A *Dictionary*
of Congenital
Malformations
and Disorders

A Dictionary of Congenital Malformations and Disorders

O. Potparic and J. Gibson

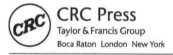

CRC Press
Taylor & Francis Group
Boca Raton London New York

CRC Press is an imprint of the
Taylor & Francis Group, an **informa** business

First published 1995 by The Parthenon Publishing Group Ltd

Published 2019 by CRC Press
Taylor & Francis Group
6000 Broken Sound Parkway NW, Suite 300
Boca Raton, FL 33487-2742

© 1995 by Taylor & Francis Group, LLC
CRC Press is an imprint of Taylor & Francis Group, an Informa business

First issued in paperback 2019

No claim to original U.S. Government works

ISBN 13: 978-0-367-44896-7 (pbk)
ISBN 13: 978-1-85070-577-2 (hbk)

Visit the Taylor & Francis Web site at
http://www.taylorandfrancis.com

and the CRC Press Web site at
http://www.crcpress.com

British Library Cataloguing in Publication Data
Potparic, O.
  Dictionary of Congenital Malformations
  and Disorders
  I. Title II. Gibson, John
  616.04303

Library of Congress Cataloging-in-Publication Data
Potparic, O. (Olivera)
  A dictionary of congenital malformations and disorders / O.
  Potparic and J. Gibson
    p. cm.
    ISBN 1-85070-577-1
    1. Genetic disorders—Dictionaries. 2. Abnormalities, Human—
  Dictionaries. I. Gibson, John. 1907-   . II. Title. III. Title.
  Congenital malformations and disorders.
    [DNLM: 1. Abnormalities—dictionaries. 2. Hereditary Diseases—
  dictionaries. QS 613 P862d 1994]
  RB155.5.P68 1994
  616.04303—dc20
  DNLM/DLC
  for Library of Congress   94-36441
                                                             CIP

Typeset by Blackpool Typesetting Services Ltd.,
Blackpool, Lancashire

Introduction

Three per cent of full-term infants are born with a congenital defect or disorder, and incidence is much higher in preterm infants and stillbirths. The defect may be a simple minor defect (such as an inguinal hernia) or a complex disorder involving many systems (such as Down syndrome). Down syndrome is the only common congenital disorder; the other defects and disorders are rare or very rare, some having been reported fewer than 20 times worldwide. The causes of most are unknown. Chromosomal defects or abnormalities are known in some. Inheritance may be autosomal dominant, autosomal recessive, or sporadic. A minor defect within the body may remain unknown throughout life if it causes no ill effects, or it may be discovered by accident or by the development of any complication. Major abnormalities and disorders can be very crippling, imposing a great strain on the patient, his or her parents, or community carers who may become responsible for the patient. Physical defects are commonly associated with mental retardation. Some physical defects may be treated surgically and some biochemical disorders may be corrected, but many disabilities can be permanent. Life span is often reduced. A number of conditions can now be detected antenatally. It is hoped that this book will be helpful in the diagnosis and understanding of them all.

A

Aagenaes syndrome

Aagenaes syndrome is due to congenital hypoplasia of lymph vessels, which causes lymphedema of the legs and recurrent cholestasis in infancy, and slow progress to hepatic cirrhosis and giant-cell hepatitis with fibrosis of the portal tracts.

Aarskog syndrome

Other name Facio–digital–genital syndrome

Aarskog syndrome is a familial X-linked disorder characterized by short stature, hypertelorism, hypoplastic maxilla, prominent umbilicus, inguinal hernia, short fingers, and cryptorchidism. The scrotum often overhangs the penis ('shawl' or 'saddleback' scrotum).

Aase syndrome

Other name Aase–Smith syndrome

Aase syndrome is probably an autosomal recessive disorder. It is characterized by intrauterine growth retardation, triphalangeal thumbs, hypoplasia of the radii, ventricular septal defect, and hypoplastic anemia. Other features can be cleft lip and palate and anomalies of clavicles and ribs.

Aase–Smith syndrome
See Aase syndrome

Absent pulmonary valve syndrome

Congenital absence of the leaflets of the pulmonary valve can occur in Fallot tetralogy or be associated with ventricular septal defect or other congenital lesions of the heart. The pulmonary arteries can be grossly dilated and can cause bronchial compression. The arterial duct is usually absent.

See also Heart malformations

N-Acetylglutamate synthetase deficiency

See Urea cycle disorders

Achard syndrome

Achard syndrome is Marfan syndrome with the addition of mandibulofacial deformities.

Achondrogenesis type I

Achondrogenesis type I is an autosomal recessive condition characterized by severe defects in the development of bone and cartilage, very small stature, large cranium, low nasal bridge, poor development of the jaws, very short limbs, and short ribs. There is imperfect ossification of many bones. Two types have been described. In type A, the proximal femurs have metaphyseal spikes and there are multiple rib fractures. In type B, the distal femurs show metaphyseal abnormalities and there are no rib fractures. Many infants are stillborn or die in the postnatal period.

Achondrogenesis type II

Other name Langer–Saldino syndrome

Achondrogenesis type II is an autosomal recessive condition characterized by cartilage abnormalities, very short stature, large cranium with large fontanels, flat nasal bridge, underdevelopment of the jaws, short limbs, short ribs without fractures, failure of ossification in several bones, and, sometimes, cleft soft palate. Most infants are stillborn or die shortly after birth.

Achondroplasia

Achondroplasia is an autosomal dominant condition and the commonest of the chondrodysplasias, with an incidence of about 1 in 26 000 live births. It is characterized by short stature, large head, small foramen magnum, slight mid-facial hypoplasia, relatively small thoracic cage, short limbs, incomplete extension of the elbow, short trident hand, small vertebral bodies, mild hypotonia, and glucose intolerance. Complications can be respiratory difficulties, hydrocephalus due to a narrow foramen magnum, and compression of the spinal cord or root due to disc lesion, kyphosis or stenosis of the spinal canal. In later life, obesity and osteoarthritis can develop, and in women, large breasts, fibroid tumors and menorrhagia can develop.

Acrocallosal syndrome

Acrocallosal syndrome is characterized by total or partial absence of the corpus callosum, craniofacial dysmorphism, polydactyly, and severe mental retardation. Other features can be retinal pigmentation anomalies, optic atrophy, strabismus, nystagmus, cleft lip and palate, cardiovascular anomalies, hernia, abnormal nipples, and fits.

Acrocephalosyndactyly type I
See Apert syndrome

Acrocephalosyndactyly type II
See Carpenter syndrome

Acrocephalosyndactyly type III
See Saethre–Chotzen syndrome

Acrodysostosis

Acrodysostosis is characterized by prenatal growth deficiency, brachycephaly, deformities of the humerus, radius and ulna, short and broad hands, hypoplastic maxilla, and mental retardation.

Acromesomelic dwarfism

Acromesomelic dwarfism is an autosomal recessive condition characterized by very short limbs, short fingers and nails, frontal prominence, and kyphosis in the lower thoracic region.

Acrorenal syndrome

Acrorenal syndrome is usually a sporadic disorder. It is characterized by hypoplastic or triphalangeal thumbs, polydactyly, malrotation of the kidneys, ureteral anomalies, and diverticulum of the bladder.

Adams–Oliver syndrome

Adams–Oliver syndrome is a variable autosomal dominant condition in which there is aplasia cutis congenita of the scalp with or without a defect of underlying skull bones and defects of the fingers and toes. Other features can be microphthalmia, cleft lip, and cryptorchidism.

Adenosine deaminase deficiency

Congenital deficiency of the enzyme adenosine deaminase is responsible for about half the cases of autosomal recessive severe combined immunodeficiency. It can also cause an immunodeficiency with a later onset and milder degree. The severe form is usually fatal within the first year of life.

See also Severe combined immunodeficiencies

Adrenal hemorrhage

Hemorrhage into the adrenal glands can be unilateral (90%) or bilateral. It can be associated with shock, hemorrhagic disorders, hypoxia, disseminated intravascular hemorrhage, or a difficult birth. The kidney is displaced downwards. Clinical features are an abdominal mass, jaundice and anemia. The condition is self-limiting, with the hematoma resolving and calcification of the area developing quickly.

Adrenal hyperplasia
See Adrenogenital syndrome

Adrenal hypoplasia

Adrenal hypoplasia can occur as a sporadic, X-linked or autosomal recessive condition, in the absence of function of the pituitary gland, as in anencephaly, and in response to lack of stimulation by adrenocorticotropic hormone (ACTH). Hypoglycemia can cause death.

Adrenal virilism
See Adrenogenital syndrome

Adrenogenital syndrome

Other names Adrenal hyperplasia; adrenal virilism

Adrenogenital syndrome may present at birth or later. It is a group of conditions in which adrenal hyperplasia is associated with a defect in the synthesis of glucocorticoids and mineral corticoids. The regulation of adrenocorticotropic hormone (ACTH) by negative feedback is interfered with and as a result the secretion of ACTH by the pituitary gland is unchecked. The highest incidence – 2.0 per 1000 live births – is in the Inuit (Eskimos). Clinical features are virilization, thickening and coarsening of the skin, acne, excessive growth of bushy hair, hyperpigmentation of the skin of the axillae, breasts, perianal region and external genitalia, hypotension, sodium retention, and hypokalemia. Male infants show pseudo-hermaphroditism (they look like females), and boys show a premature growth of pubic and axillary hair, male-type alopecia of the scalp, enlarged penis, and increased folding of the scrotal skin. Female infants show masculinization. Women have primary amenorrhea, enlarged clitoris, failure of breast development, acne, excess hair, and increased muscular development. Adult men show little change in normal appearance and development.

Adrenoleukodystrophy

Congenital adrenoleukodystrophy, an X-linked autosomal recessive condition occurring in both sexes, can present at birth with adrenal insufficiency, craniofacial anomalies, and anomalies of the central nervous system.

AEC syndrome

Other name Hay–Wells syndrome

AEC syndrome is an autosomal syndrome characterized by:
A – ankylopharon (adhesion of the ciliary edges of the eyelids to each other);
E – ectodermal defects; and
C – cleft lip and sometimes also cleft palate.
Associated features can be absent or dystrophic nails, sparse wire-like hair or alopecia, pointed and widely spaced teeth, a broad bridge to the nose, recessed maxilla, decreased sweating, and, sometimes, ventricular septal defect, patent ductus arteriosus, and deafness.

Afzelius syndrome
See Immotile cilia syndrome

Aglossia congenita

Aglossia congenita is a congenital absence of the tongue.

Agranulocytosis
See Kostmann syndrome

Agyria-pachygyria

Agyria–pachygyria is a group of disorders of cortical neuronal migration due either to a primary agenesis or to a secondary destruction at an early stage of formation. In pachygyria, there is evidence of some primary and secondary gyration. The most extreme form is lissencephaly, in which the surface of the brain is smooth, without gyri or sulci.

See also Lissencephaly

Aicardi syndrome

Aicardi syndrome is an X-linked disorder characterized by agenesis of the corpus callosum, chorioretinal lacunae, vertebral anomalies, fits, mental retardation, and, sometimes, multiple papillomas of the choroid plexus.

Alagille syndrome

Other name Syndromatic bile duct paucity

Alagille syndrome is an autosomal dominant disorder characterized by cholestasis, hypercholesterolemia, neonatal jaundice, prominent forehead and chin, bulbous nose, peripheral pulmonary stenosis, vertebral defects, and, sometimes, atrial and ventricular septal defect, patent ductus arteriosus, and coarctation of the aorta.

Albinism
See Oculocutaneous albinism

Albright syndrome

Other names Polyostotic fibrous dysplasia; McCune–Albright syndrome

Albright syndrome is characterized by osteitis fibrosa disseminata (a fibrous dysplasia of several bones which can induce pathological fractures) and melanotic macules in the skin, present at birth or appearing in neonatal life, usually unilateral and seen especially on the forehead, the back of the neck, the sacral region, and the buttocks. Other features can be endocrine dysfunction and precocious puberty.

Alexander syndrome

Alexander syndrome is an autosomal recessive condition which presents in infantile, juvenile and adult forms. It is characterized by leukodystrophy, megalencephaly, and normal or enlarged cerebral ventricles. Infants affected are likely to die between 5 months and 5 years.

Ambras syndrome

Ambras syndrome is an autosomal dominant condition characterized by the whole body being covered by fine long hair (except areas in which normally no hair grows), dysmorphic facies, absence of teeth, and retarded first and second dentitions.

Amniotic band syndrome

Amniotic band syndrome is due to the formation of amniotic bands between the fetus and a sticky chorion, due to the loss of some amnion early in pregnancy. There is an increased risk in Ehlers–Danlos syndrome and Marfan syndrome. By constricting the limbs, these bands can cause edema beyond the constriction, terminal syndactyly and limb amputation.

Amyoplasia congenita disruptive sequence

See Arthrogryposis multiplex congenita

Amniotic fluid α-fetoprotein

The α-fetoprotein level is raised in neural tube defects, and may be raised in bowel atresia, bladder exstrophy, congenital nephrosis, (Finnish type), focal dermal hypoplasia and other skin defects, gastroschisis, Meckel syndrome, omphalocele, sacrococcygeal teratoma, spontaneous intrauterine death, and Turner syndrome.

Anal malformations

Anal malformations occur in about 1 in 5000 births. Males are slightly more commonly affected than females. Associated abnormalities are vertebral malformations, genitourinary malformations, and other gastrointestinal malformations.

Anal agenesis is a failure of the anus to develop. The normal site of the anus can be marked by a dimple. The clinical features are absence of the anus and a failure to pass meconium.

Anal agenesis with fistula is anal agenesis with an ectopic opening of the anus (the so-called fistula). In males, the opening is usually into the perineum; it can be into the urethra. In females, it is into the vulva or perineum.

Anal stenosis is a narrowing of the anal canal, with difficulty in passing feces, which can be ribbon-shaped.

Imperforate anal membrane is an epithelial membrane above the anal opening. It has no aperture and the infant fails to pass meconium.

Anderson-Fabry syndrome
See Fabry syndrome

Anencephaly

Anencephaly is an absence of the cranial vault and a failure of development of the cerebral hemispheres. The cerebellum can be absent or rudimentary, the hypothalamus is malformed, and the internal carotid arteries are hypoplastic. Spina bifida is commonly present. Other features can be cardiovascular abnormalities and small adrenal glands. About 75–80% of sufferers are stillborn; survivors are likely to die within a few hours or weeks of life. Prenatal diagnosis can be made by measurement of the maternal serum α-fetoprotein, which is raised in this condition and in spina bifida.

Angelman syndrome
See Happy puppet syndrome

Angiokeratoma corporis diffusum
See Fabry syndrome

Aniridia-Wilms tumor syndrome

Aniridia is congenital absence of the iris. Aniridia–Wilms tumor syndrome may show an interstitial defect of the lip, but this is not found in all patients. Other features can be microcephaly, growth deficiency, badly developed ears, congenital cataract, nystagmus, ptosis, blindness, hypospadias, cryptorchidism, and mental retardation.

Ankyloglossia inferior

Other name Tongue-tie

Ankyloglossia inferior is a short frenulum which interferes with the movements of the tongue. If it does not inferfere with sucking and swallowing, it need not be cut, as it can be expected to lengthen in time.

Ankyloglossia superior

Ankyloglossia superior is an attachment of the tongue to the roof of the mouth. It is a rare condition and can be associated with macroglossia, micrognathia, and cleft palate.

Anophthalmia

Anophthalmia is congenital absence of the eyes or the presence of vestigial eyes. It can occur without other congenital abnormalities, but in 40–73% of cases other malformations are present. It can be due to fetal damage occurring up to the time of mid-pregnancy and to genetic, chromosomal and environmental causes; a genetic etiology is suspected in most cases. Environmental causes can be drugs, infections, and toxins. It has been attributed to antenatal exposure to vitamin A, thalidomide, ethambutol, lysergide, congenital varicella, rubella, influenza, and parvovirus B19 infection.

Anterior cleavage syndrome

Other name Mesodermal dysgenesis

Anterior cleavage syndrome is an anomalous development of the anterior segment of the eye, with corneal opacities, an abnormal anterior-chamber angle defect, abnormalities of the iris, and glaucoma.

Antimongoloid syndrome

Antimongoloid syndrome is a congenital disorder due to partial deletion of chromosome 21. It is characterized by an antimongoloid slant of the eyes, craniodysmorphism, retarded skeletal growth, undescended testes, hypospadias, and mental retardation.

Antley–Bixler syndrome

Other name Multisynostotic osteodysgenesis

Antley–Bixler syndrome is characterized by craniosynostosis, brachycephaly, mid-facial hypoplasia, choanal stenosis, joint contractures, radiohumeral synostosis, arachnodactyly, and femoral bowing and fractures.

Aortic coarctation

Coarctation of the aorta is usually situated just beyond the origin of the left subclavian artery. Pulses proximal to the lesion are stronger than those distal to it; the pulses and blood pressure in the arms are greater than those in the legs. A systolic murmur may be heard posteriorly over the site of the coarctation. The undersurfaces of the ribs may be notched by tortuous intercostal arteries.

Aortic interrupted arch

Aortic interrupted arch is a lack of connection between the ascending and descending aorta. The discontinuity may be distal to the left subclavian artery, distal to the left common carotid artery, or distal to the innominate artery. After birth, blood can pass into the descending aorta through the ductus arteriosus, but this ceases when the ductus closes, which it usually does. Clinical features are the development of congestive heart failure and, as the ductus arteriosus closes, of lack of pulses and mottling in the lower half of the body. Cardiac malformations are common complications.

Aortic stenosis

Aortic stenosis may be *valvular* with fusion of the two leaflets of unequal size, *subaortic*, due to a tunnel-type obstruction, a fibromuscular membrane or hypertrophic cardiomyopthy, or *supraclavicular* and part of the supraclavicular syndrome (elfin face, mental retardation, friendly personality, and sometimes hypercalcemia). The ascending aorta may be dilated above the stenosis.

See also Heart malformations

Apert syndrome

Other name Acrocephalosyndactyly type I

Apert syndrome is an autosomal dominant condition characterized by oxycephaly (a congenital deformity of the head which rises to a peak) associated with syndactyly and mental retardation. Other features can be hypertelorism, strabismus, proptosis, downward slanting of the palpebral fissures, low-set ears, submucous cleft palate, malocclusion of the teeth, and a ventricular septal defect.

Aplasia cutis congenita

Aplasia cutis congenita is localized congenital absence of skin. The cause is unknown. Both autosomal dominant and autosomal recessive transmission can occur. The patches can be on the scalp, trunk and limbs. Associated conditions can be cleft lip and palate, congenital heart disease, cerebral malformations, and clubbing of the hands and feet.

Apple peel syndrome

Apple peel syndrome is a congenital condition in which the superior mesenteric artery causes an obstruction to the jejunum, with vomiting of bile and intestinal obstruction in neonatal life. The coils of intestine wrapped round the artery have been compared to apple peel.

Arginine vasopressin deficiency

Congenital arginine vasopressin deficiency is a rare disorder, which is sometimes associated with disorders of the central nervous system. Polyuria is the clinical feature.

Argininosuccinic acidemia
See Urea cycle disorders

Arteriovenous fistula

Arteriovenous fistula is a direct connection between an artery and vein, bypassing capillaries, or an angioma with arterial and venous connections. After birth, the right and left sides of the heart can become overloaded, the heart is unable to cope with the venous return, and heart failure develops.

Arthrogryposis multiplex congenita

Other names Arthromyodysplasia; amyoplasia congenita disruptive sequence; myodystrophia fetalis deformans

Arthrogryposis multiplex congenita presents *in utero* with decreased movements. Birth can be difficult and breech presentation can occur. The principal feature is contractures of joints. The shoulders are internally rotated. Elbows are fixed in extension; the wrists and hands are held in flexion. The metacarpophalangeal joints are fixed in severe flexion and the interphalangeal joints are slightly flexed. The hips may be dislocated. There is decreased growth of the limbs. Other features can be bowel atresia, trunk muscle defects, hernias, and torticollis.

Arthromyodysplasia
See Arthrogryposis multiplex congenita

Article V syndrome

Article V syndrome is characterized by anomalies that are:
A – anal
R – renal
T – tracheal
I – intestinal
C – cardiac
L – limb
E – esophageal
V – vertebral (sometimes)

Asphyxiating thoracic dysplasia
See Jeune syndrome

Asplenia syndrome

Other name Ivemark syndrome

Asplenia syndrome is a congenital syndrome characterized by absence of the spleen, transposition of the viscera, transposition of the great arteries, and congenital heart defects. The etiology is unknown. Death occurs at an early age.

Ataxia–telangiectasia syndrome

Ataxia–telangiectasia syndrome is an autosomal recessive disorder with an incidence of 2–3 per 100 000 live births. Clinical features are ataxia, telangiectasia, chronic sinus and pulmonary diseases, variable B-cell and T-cell deficiencies, and endocrine abnormalities. The ataxia is progressive and is due to progressive degeneration of neurons of the cerebellar cortex. It is usually the presenting feature and becomes apparent when the child starts to walk. Other neurological features are progressive muscular weakness, choreo-athetosis, intention tremor, nystagmus, dysarthria, and a failure of intellectual development over the age of 9 years. The telangiectasia appears in the conjunctiva, nose, ears and shoulders. Other skin anomalies are atrophy of the skin, premature graying of the hair, vitiligo or cafe-au-lait spots, multiple keratoses, and basal cell carcinoma. T-cell deficiency causes lymphopenia; B-cell deficiency causes absence of immunoglobulin (Ig) A and IgE. Endocrinological defects are hypoplasia of the ovaries, cytoplasmic vacuoles in the anterior pituitary and elevated gonadotropin levels. Recurrent infections are common. The prognosis is poor, with death usually due to pneumonia or bronchiectasis.

Atelosteogenesis
See Giant cell chondrodysplasia

Atrial septal defect

Atrial septal defect is a congenital condition which may not produce symptoms in infancy. The defect may be a sinus venosus defect, a primum atrial defect, or a secundum atrial defect. Symptoms in childhood are fatigue and dyspnea on exertion; there may be a prominent right cardiac impulse and palpable pulmonary pulsation.

See also Heart malformations

Auriculo-osteodysplasia syndrome
See Beals syndrome

Axenfield syndrome

Axenfield syndrome is an autosomal dominant condition characterized by iris abnormalities, glaucoma, and posterior embryotoxon (a congenital opaque marginal corneal ring).

B

Baller-Gerold syndrome

Other name Craniosynostosis–radial aplasia syndrome

Baller–Gerold syndrome is an autosomal recessive condition characterized by craniosynostosis, hypoplasia or absence of a radius, missing carpals, metacarpals and phalanges, hypoplastic or absent thumbs, bifid uvula, anteriorly placed or imperforate anus, growth retardation, and mental retardation.

Bardet-Biedl syndrome

Bardet–Biedl syndrome is an autosomal recessive disorder characterized by obesity, polydactyly and/or syndactyly, retinitis pigmentosa, hypogonadism, and mental retardation.

Barlow syndrome
See Prolapsed mitral valve syndrome

Basal cell nevus syndrome
See Gorlin syndrome

Bat ear
See External ear disorders

Beals syndrome

Other name Contractural arachnodactyly; auriculo-osteodysplasia syndrome

Beals syndrome is an autosomal dominant disorder characterized by arachnodactyly, limited extension of elbows and knees, joint contracture of fingers, elbows, knees and hips, and crumpled ears. Other features can be congenital heart disease, kyphosis, scoliosis, or kyphoscoliosis. The clinical features overlap with those of Marfan syndrome. Mild expression can produce crumpled ears, camptodactyly, adducted thumbs, limited elbow or knee extension, kyphosis, scoliosis or kyphoscoliosis, hypoplasia of calf muscles, and congenital heart disease.

Beckwith syndrome
See Beckwith-Wiedemann syndrome

Beckwith-Wiedemann syndrome

Other names Beckwith syndrome; visceromegaly syndrome

Beckwith-Wiedemann syndrome is an autosomal dominant condition characterized by high birth weight, omphalocele, macroglossia, hepatomegaly, splenomegaly, hyperplasia of the kidney, congenital abnormalities of the urinary tract, slight microcephaly, and a susceptibility to develop benign and malignant tumors, especially rhabdomyosarcoma and Wilms tumor. Pancreatic island-cell hyperplasia can cause hyperinsulinemia and hypoglycemia. The infant can show an excessive response to intravenous glucose, which results in further hypoglycemia. The liability to develop hypoglycemia is usually lost as the infant becomes older.

Benign congenital hypotonia

Benign congenital hypotonia is a form of congenital myopathy in which the hypotonia either remains about the same or gradually disappears.

Benign congenital neutropenia

Benign congenital neutropenia is generally a harmless condition in which the granulocyte count is less than 1500 cells/μl. The blood is otherwise normal. Severe infections are unlikely.

Berardinelli syndrome

Berardinelli syndrome is an autosomal recessive disorder and an inborn error of metabolism of which the defect is unknown. It is characterized by general lipodystrophy, accelerated growth and maturation, muscle hypertrophy, coarse skin, hirsutism, enlarged liver, large penis, hyperlipemia, hyperinsulinism, and hyperglucagonemia. Cirrhosis of the liver can be a complication.

Bickers-Adams syndrome

Bickers-Adams syndrome is an X-linked stenosis of the cerebral aqueduct, which causes hydrocephalus.

BIDS syndrome

BIDS syndrome is an autosomal recessive inherited disease characterized by:
B – brittle hair
I – impairment, mental and physical
D – decreased fertility
S – short stature

See also IBIDS syndrome

Biliary atresia

Atresia of the bile ducts can occur both within and outside the liver. The cause is unknown. It is not known to be familial or inherited. It can be associated with congenital cytomegalovirus infection, congenital rubella, and prenatal *Listeria monocytogenes* infection. The ducts may be partly or completely absent or stenotic. The most prominent clinical features are persistent jaundice and absence of bile in the stools. The liver becomes enlarged and firm and the spleen enlarges as portal hyertension develops. Death is inevitable if the fault cannot be surgically corrected or the child cannot receive a liver transplant.

Binder syndrome

Other name Maxillonasal dysplasia

Binder syndrome is a congenital disorder characterized by hypoplasia of the maxilla, prognathism of the lower jaw, agenesis of the nasal septum, and flattening of the nose. Other features can be cleft palate, dental abnormalities, cervical vertebral malformations, and mental retardation. It is usually sporadic but can be familial.

Bird-headed dwarfism
See Seckel syndrome

Bixler syndrome
See HMC syndrome

Bjornstad syndrome

Bjornstad syndrome is an autosomal dominant inherited condition of pili torti (twisted hair) associated with nerve deafness.

Bladder exstrophy

Bladder exstrophy is a congenital deficiency of the bladder and anterior abdominal wall. The anterior abdominal wall is replaced by the undeveloped anterior wall of the bladder, with exposure of the ureteral orifices and trigone and dribbling of urine from the mucosal surface. The incidence is 1 in 30 000 births. The male : female ratio is 2 : 1. In males, the penis shows epispadias and the testes are usually undescended. In females, the labia are widely separated, the clitoris can fail to fuse or be fissured, and the vagina can be absent, dislocated anteriorly, or replaced by a rectovaginal cloaca. Inguinal hernia can be present.

Bland–Garland syndrome

Bland–Garland syndrome is left-ventricular failure due to the left coronary artery arising from the pulmonary artery and not from the aorta. If the syndrome is untreated, death is likely in childhood or adolescence.

Blepharophimosis

Blepharophimosis is an autosomal dominant condition characterized by phimosis of the eyelids, ptosis, fibrosis of the levator palpebrae muscle, poorly developed ears, and hypogonadism. Cardiac defects may be present. Intelligence is usually low to normal.

Type I is an autosomal dominant condition which occurs in females only. The females are infertile. Type II is less common. It is an autosomal dominant condition with incomplete penetrance and occurs in males and females.

Bloch–Sulzberger syndrome

Other name Incontinentia pigmenti

Bloch–Sulzberger syndrome is probably due to a single mutant gene. It occurs mainly in females. A vesiculobullous eruption is present at birth or develops within 2 weeks; development can occur later in life. From the 12th week of life, hyperpigmentation of the skin develops, especially in the lateral regions of the trunk and in the perimammary areas. After the age of 2 years, the pigmentation begins to fade. Other features can be cataracts, strabismus, optic nerve atrophy, blue sclerae, scarring alopecia, spoon-shaped nails, short stature, spina bifida, cleft lip and palate, microcephaly, spastic paralysis, hydrocephalus, teeth and ear abnormalities, cardiac abnormalities, and mental retardation. Over 15% of patients become blind.

Bloom syndrome

Bloom syndrome is an autosomal recessive inherited condition most common in Ashkenazi Jews. There is a defect in DNA replication. It is characterized by low birth weight, short stature, dolicocephalic skull, characteristic facies with a narrow prominent nose, a receding chin and hypoplastic malar region, telangiectatic erythema of the face, and photosensitivity. Café-au-lait spots are present in about half the patients. Multiple severe infections of the gastrointestinal tract and respiratory tract are common. There is an increased incidence of leukemia, lymphoma, lymphosarcoma, and carcinoma of the mouth and gastrointestinal tract. Sexual development is normal, but males are infertile, owing to sperm defects. The intelligence is usually normal, and neurological abnormalities are unusual. Immunoglobulin levels are low and chromosomal abnormalities of various kinds are present.

Blue rubber bleb nevus syndrome

Blue rubber bleb nevus syndrome is an autosomal dominant inherited condition in which there are blue cavernous hemangiomas in the skin. They are about 3–4 cm in diameter and feel like rubber. They can be painful. Excessive sweating can occur. Similar hemangiomas are present in the gastrointestinal tract and can, by bleeding, cause melena.

Börjeson–Forssman–Lehmann syndrome

Börjeson–Forssman–Lehmann syndrome is an X-linked recessive syndrome characterized by microcephaly, coarse facies, large ears, nystagmus, ptosis, optic nerve abnormalities, retinal abnormalities, neuronal migration abnormalities in the brain, hypogonadism, severe mental retardation, and obesity in later life.

Bourneville syndrome
See Tuberous sclerosis

Brachmann-de Lange syndrome
See Cornelia de Lange syndrome

Brachydactyly

Brachydactyly, as an isolated bilateral condition, is usually autosomal dominant. Conditions in which it is a feature include Albright's hereditary osteodystrophy, pseudohypoparathyroidism and Turner syndrome.

Brachydactyly syndrome type E

Brachydactyly syndrome type E (Bell's classification) is an autosomal dominant condition characterized by short metacarpals and metatarsals, short phalanges, and prenatal growth deficiency.

Branchial cysts

Other names Branchiogenic cysts; lateral cervical cysts; cervical thymic cysts

Branchial cysts arise in the embryo from the pharyngeal pouch, thymic stalk, or branchial groove. They can be congenital or appear later in life. They appear behind the sternomastoid muscle and may project in front of its anterior margin. They are liable to become infected and filled with pus.

Branchiogenic cysts
See Branchial cysts

Branchio-oculofacial syndrome
See Hematogenous branchial cleft syndrome

Branchio-otorenal syndrome

Other name Melnick–Fraser syndrome

Branchio-otorenal syndrome is an autosomal dominant condition characterized by deafness, preauricular pits, branchial cysts or fistulae, malformation of the external, middle and inner ear, lacrimal duct aplasia or stenosis, and developmental malformations or agenesis of the kidneys. The syndrome occurs in about 2% of severely deaf children.

Broad thumb syndrome
See Rubinstein–Taybi syndrome

Brown syndrome

Brown syndrome is the occurrence of an inferior oblique palsy of the 'eye in a patient with rheumatoid arthritis. It is thought to be due to a tenosynovitis of the tendon sheath of the superior oblique muscle of the eye. The palsy can be intermittent and accompanied by clicking in the region of the trochlea.

Brusa-Torricelli syndrome

Brusa–Torricelli syndrome is an association of aniridia (congenital absence of the iris) and other congenital defects with neuroblastoma.

Bulldog syndrome

Bulldog syndrome is an X-linked congenital condition characterized by a large square protruding lower jaw, a broad nasal bridge, an upturned tip of the nose, macroglossia, and broad short limbs, and this form is said to resemble a bulldog.

Bullous ichthyosiform erythroderma

Other name Epidermolytic hyperkeratosis

Bullous ichthyosiform erythroderma is an autosomal dominant skin condition which may be present at birth. It is characterized by erythroderma, scaling and bullae.

C

C1 deficiency

C1 is the first component of complement and is composed of the three glycoproteins C1q, C1r and C1s. Deficiency of C1 can be inherited or acquired and is likely to cause symptoms similar to those of systemic lupus erythematosus and susceptibility to recurrent infections.

C1 inhibitor deficiency

C1 inhibitor is a member of the serpin family of protease inhibitors. Hereditary angioneurotic edema occurs in people who are heterozygous for C1 inhibitor deficiency. Hereditary angioneurotic edema is characterized by recurrent acute attacks of the skin and mucosa. Edema of the skin is not painful, does not itch and is non-pitting; erythematous mottling can be present. Organs likely to be affected are the larynx and gastrointestinal tract. The onset is usually in childhood and attacks usually last for 24–72 h.

C3 syndrome

Other names Cranio-cerebello-cardiac dysplasia; Ritscher–Schinzel syndrome

C3 syndrome is an autosomal recessive condition characterized by hindbrain malformations, ventricular septal defect with parachute-shaped mitral valve, micronychia (small nails), and hypoplasia of the terminal phalanges.

C4 inherited deficiency

C4 is the fourth component of complement, a three-chain glycoprotein and a major protein in the classical pathway of complement activation. Complete C4 deficiency gives rise in most cases to systemic lupus erythematosus, discoid lupus erythematosus and an increased susceptibility to infections. Partial C4 deficiency predisposes to different autoimmune diseases, including systemic lupus erythematosus, discoid lupus erythematosus, systemic sclerosis, IgA deficiency, IgA nephropathy, Henoch–Schönlein purpura, chronic active hepatitis, Gougerot–Sjögren disease, common variable immunodeficiency, subacute sclerosing panencephalitis, and benign recurrent hematuria.

C6, C7, C8, C9 deficiencies

Inherited deficiencies of the terminal components (C6, C7, C8, C9) of complement can be associated with neisserial infections and possibly sometimes with other infections.

Caffey pseudo-Hurler syndrome
See Generalized gangliosidosis syndrome

Camptomelic dysplasia

Camptomelic dysplasia (*camptomelique* – bent limb) is an autosomal recessive condition characterized by bowed tibiae, flat facies, growth deficiency, large brain, short flat vertebrae, hypoplastic scapulae, cleft palate, and, sometimes, cardiac defects and hydramnios. Death in the postnatal period is common.

Camurati-Engelmann syndrome

Camurati–Engelmann syndrome is a familial dominant disorder characterized by fusiform enlargement of the shafts of the bones of the legs, other bone deformities, eye defects, and hypogonadism.

Canavan syndrome

Canavan syndrome is an autosomal recessive inherited disease in which a spongy degeneration of the white matter of the brain develops in infancy and causes optic atrophy with blindness, muscle rigidity, poor head control, and exaggerated reflexes. The head can become enlarged. Death occurs in the first 5 years of life.

Cantrell pentalogy

Cantrell pentalogy is an association of cleft sternum, lower thoracic wall malformation, diaphragmatic defect, cardiac anomaly and pericardial defect. Omphalocele is an associated condition.

Capillary telangiectasia
See Intracranial capillary angioma

Carbamyl phosphate synthetase deficiency
See Urea cycle disorders

Cardioauditory syndrome
See Jervell–Lange–Nielsen syndrome

Cardio–facio–cutaneous syndrome

Other name Noonan-like short stature syndrome

Cardio–facio–cutaneous syndrome is an autosomal dominant condition with a variable phenotypic expression. It is characterized by short stature, cardiac anomalies (atrial septal aneurysm, hypertrophic cardiomyopathy), macrocephaly, facial anomalies (roundness, hypertelorism, broad nose, sparse eyebrows), and cutaneous anomalies (hyperkeratosis, erythematous plaques on the cheeks and trunk).

Carpenter syndrome

Other name Acrocephalosyndactyly type II

Carpenter syndrome is a congenital syndrome characterized by acrocephaly, sometimes of severe degree, premature closing of the cranial sutures, hypertelorism, a flat nasal bridge, and a hypoplastic mandible. Webbing of digits three and four is present; there may be abnormalities of the toes. Other features can be short neck, omphalocele, pulmonary stenosis, atrial ventricular defect, or Fallot tetralogy.

Cartilage–hair hypoplasia syndrome
See Metaphyseal chondrodysplasia, McKusick type

Cartilage–hair hypoplasia with immunodeficiency

Cartilage–hair hypoplasia can be associated with immunodeficiency, inherited as an autosomal recessive trait and varying in intensity from mild dysfunction to severe combined immunodeficiency. It can develop early in childhood or after a few years.

Cataract

Congenital cataract occurs in about 1 in 250 births. Several forms of inheritance can exist, with most genetic forms without a metabolic cause having a dominant inheritance, with the risk for sibs of about 10% and the risk for offspring of an affected person just below 50%. Cataracts are commonly associated with chromosomal disorders, especially of chromosomes 13, 18, and 21. Others occur in metabolic disorders, especially galactosemia, in congenital ichthyosis, and in ectodermal dysplasias. Other causes are maternal rubella and Turner syndrome.

Cataract-oligophrenia syndrome
See Marinesco–Sjögren syndrome

Catel-Manzke syndrome

Catel–Manzke syndrome is Pierre Robin syndrome with abnormalities of the index and little fingers and atrial or ventricular septal defects.

Cat-eye syndrome

Other name Schmid–Fraccaro syndrome

Cat-eye syndrome is an autosomal dominant condition, most cases having one or more extra copies of chromosome fragment 22q11. Clinical features are a vertical coloboma of the iris (hence 'cat eye'), downward-slanting palpebral fissures, preauricular fistula, anal atresia, umbilical hernia, cardiac and renal defects, and mental retardation.

Caudal dysplasia
See Caudal regression syndrome

Caudal regression syndrome

Other names Caudal dysplasia; sacral agenesis

Caudal regression syndrome is characterized by maldevelopment of the sacrum, coccyx, and lumbar vetebrae, absence of the body of the sacrum, failure of normal development of the lower end of the spinal cord and related spinal roots and nerves, incontinence of urine and feces, impaired development of the lower limbs, popliteal webs limiting movement of the knees, and talipes equinovarus. Associated conditions can be microcephaly, meningocele, cleft lip and palate, renal agenesis and imperforate anus. The cause is unknown. Most cases are sporadic. There is an association with diabetes mellitus, with about one child in 350 of diabetic mothers suffering from caudal regression syndrome.

Cenani–Lenz syndactyly syndrome

Cenani–Lenz syndactyly syndrome is an autosomal recessive condition characterized by syndactyly of fingers, radioulnar synostosis, shortened forearms, hypoplasia of the phalanges, and sometimes syndactyly of the toes.

Centromeric region syndrome

Centromeric region syndrome is an immunodeficiency syndrome in which there is chromosomal instability, breakage, and unusual configurations, especially on chromosomes 1, 9, and 16. The immunodeficiency is variable. There is a low production of immunoglobulin. Clinical features are likely to be ataxia, dystonia, choreoathetosis, dysmorphic facies, bilateral epicanthic folds, exomphalos, recurrent respiratory infections, failure to thrive and growth retardation.

Cerebral gigantism
See Sotos syndrome

Cerebro–costo–mandibular syndrome

Cerebro–costo–mandibular syndrome may be an autosomal recessive or an autosomal dominant condition. It is characterized by intrauterine growth retardation, rib abnormalities, severe micrognathia, tracheal cartilaginous ring abnormalities, small thorax, respiratory insufficiency, vertebral abnormalities, and mental retardation. Many affected infants die in the first year of life.

Cerebro–facio–thoracic dysplasia

Cerebro–facio–thoracic dysplasia is probably an autosomal recessive condition. It is characterized by facial abnormalities, multiple abnormalities of the vertebrae and ribs, and mental retardation.

Cerebro-hepato-renal syndrome

See Zellweger syndrome

Cerebro-oculo-facial-skeletal syndrome

Other name COFS syndrome

Cerebro-oculo-facial-skeletal syndrome is an autosomal recessive condition characterized by microcephaly, reduction in cerebral white matter, small lower jaw, flexor contractures, hypotonia, cataracts, and narrowing of the palpebral fissures. The course is downhill, growth is poor, cachexia develops, and death, usually due to pulmonary infection, is likely to occur within the first 5 years of life.

Cervical thymic cysts

See Branchial cysts

Cervico-oculo-acoustic syndrome

Other name Wildervanck syndrome

Cervico-oculo-acoustic syndrome occurs almost exclusively in females, but the pattern of inheritance is unknown. It consists of a triad: (a) Klippel–Feil anomaly (fused cervical vertebrae); (b) Douane anomaly (adducens nerve palsy with retractio bulbi; and (c) congenital sensorineural deafness.

CHARGE syndrome

Other name Pagon syndrome

CHARGE syndrome is a congenital disorder characterized by:
C - coloboma
H - heart defects
A - atresia choanae
R - retardation, mental and physical
G - genitourinary anomalies
E - ear anomalies and deafness
Other features can be microphthalmos, facial palsy, orofacial clefts, and tracheo-esophageal atresia or fistula.

Chediak–Higashi syndrome

Chediak–Higashi syndrome is a multisystem autosomal recessive inherited disorder (described separately by Chediak in Cuba and Higashi in Japan). Peroxidase-positive lysosomal granules are present in granulocytes and giant granules in Schwann cells and other tissues. Clinical features are oculocutaneous albinism with depigmentation of the hair, skin and retina, recurrent bacterial infections, strabismus, nystagmus, and photophobia. Staphylococcal, streptococcal and fungal infections of the respiratory tract and skin occur in early childhood; later there can be fits, an enlarged liver and spleen, jaundice, enlarged hilar lymph nodes, gingivitis and pseudomembranous sloughing of the buccal membrane. At about 5–6 years of age, a progressive neuropathy is liable to involve cranial and peripheral nerves. Lymphoreticular malignancy can be a complication. Death usually occurs in childhood or the teens, and usually from an infection.

Chest wall congenital deformities

Deformities of the sternum are characterized by agenesis, bifid sternum, pectus carinatum, and pectus excavatum. There can be absence of one or more ribs, fusion of ribs, or cervical rib.

Deformities of the spine can include hemivertebrae, scoliosis, and Sprengel deformity. Pectoral muscles can be absent.

Chilaiditi syndrome
See Intestinal hepatodiaphragmatic interposition

Child syndrome

CHILD syndrome is an X-linked congenital condition characterized by:
CD – congenital dysplasia
I   – ichthyosiform erythroderma
LD – limb deformity
Other features are hypoplasia of paired organs and unilateral ichthyosis. The male : female ratio is 19 : 1; the condition is fatal in males.

Choanal atresia

Congenital atresia of the posterior nares is a rare condition caused by persistence of the bucconasal membrane. It occurs equally in males and females. Unilateral atresia may not be apparent in the neonate, but bilateral atresia causes respiratory obstruction, cyanosis and asphyxia. It can be associated with congenital abnormalities of the iris, ear, heart, esophagus and digits, and is a feature of Treacher Collins syndrome, CHARGE syndrome, and glossoptosis-apnea syndrome.

Choledochal cyst

Choledochal cyst is a congenital cystic dilatation of the common bile duct, and can be due to a congenital defect of the duct wall, an abnormal passage of the duct through the duodenal wall, or a mucosal valve in the duct. It is usually symptomless, but it is occasionally a cause of obstructive jaundice.

Chondrodysplasia
See Ollier syndrome

Chondrodysplasia punctata, Conradi–Hünermann type

The Conradi-Hünermann type of chondrodysplasia is an autosomal dominant condition characterized by asymmetric shortening of long bones, joint contractures, flat face, short nose with depressed bridge, cataracts (20% of cases), and alopecia or atrophic skin changes.

Chondrodystrophic myotonia
See Schwartz–Jampel syndrome

Chondroectodermal dysplasia
See Ellis–van Creveld syndrome

Chondrodysplasia punctata, rhizomelic type

The rhizomelic type of chondrodysplasia punctata is an autosomal recessive condition characterized by rhizomelic joint contractures, short nose with depressed bridge, flat face, cataracts, ichthyosiform erythroderma, mental retardation, and failure to thrive. Death in the first year of life is likely.

Christian syndrome

Christian syndrome is an autosomal dominant condition characterized by short thumbs and distal phalanges.

Chromosome 4, short-arm deletion syndrome

Other name Wolf–Hirschhorn syndrome

Chromosome 4, short-arm deletion syndrome is characterized by growth deficiency of prenatal onset, microcephaly, hypertelorism, epicanthic folds, iris deformity, cleft lip or palate, cardiac abnormalities, hypospadias, cryptorchidism, fits, severe mental retardation, and other abnormalities.

Chromosome 8p deletion syndrome

Chromosome 8p deletion syndrome is due to partial deletion of the short arm of chromosome 8. It is characterized by dysmorphic facies, congenital heart defects, mental retardation, and postnatal growth retardation.

Chromosome 9p deletion syndrome

Chromosome 9p deletion syndrome is due to deletion of the distal portion of the short arm of chromosome 9, and is characterized by craniostenosis, triagonocephalic configuration of the skull, upslanting palpebral fissures, short neck, cardiac abnormalities (patent ductus arteriosus, ventricular septal defect, pulmonary stenosis), and severe mental abnormalities. Growth is usually normal.

Chromosome partial 10q syndrome

Chromosome partial 10q syndrome is characterized by growth deficiency of prenatal origin, microcephaly, dysmorphic facies, cleft palate, cardiac, renal, ocular and cerebral abnormalities, and severe mental retardation, with about one half of the patients dying within the first year of life.

Chromosome 13q deletion syndrome

Chromosome 13q deletion syndrome is due to deletion of band 14 in the long arm of chromosome 13. It is characterized principally by prenatal growth deficiency and mental retardation. Other features that are sometimes present are microcephaly, retinoblastoma, short neck and webbing of the neck, small or absent thumbs, short big toe, cardiac defects, hypospadias, cryptorchidism, and focal lumbar agenesis.

Chromosome 18p deletion syndrome

Chromosome 18p deletion syndrome is due to either deletion of the short arm of chromosome 18 or a deficiency in a ring 18 chromosome. It is characterized by ptosis, epicanthic folds, hypertelorism, small hands and feet, growth deficiency, and mental retardation. Other features can be IgA absence or deficiency, cataracts, strabismus, webbed neck, congenital dislocation of the hip, inguinal hernia, and features similar to rheumatoid arthritis.

Chromosome 18q deletion syndrome

Chromosome 18q deletion syndrome is an autosomal deletion syndrome characterized by brachycephaly, facial dysmorphism, congenital heart abnormalities, genital hypoplasia, and abnormalities of the toes.

Chromosome 21q deletion syndrome

Chromosome 21q deletion syndrome is due to deletion of the distal arm of chromosome 21 and shows characteristic facial features, blindness and mental retardation.

Chronic granulomatous disease

Chronic granulomatous disease is an inherited group of disorders in which phagocytic leukocytes (eosinophils, neutrophils, macrophages and monocytes) fail to undergo a 'respiratory burst' when stimulated. Normally, the products of the respiratory burst, which include hypochlorous acid and superoxide, have an important role in killing pathogenic micro-organisms, parasites and fungi. In the majority of families, the disease is transmitted as an X-chromosome-linked trait (X-CGD) in chromosome position Xp.21.1. At least three genetically distinct forms of autosomal recessive disease have been reported. The patient suffers severe infections and can die in infancy.

Chylothorax

Congenital chylothorax is due to intrauterine obstruction of the thoracic duct. It can occur alone or in association with other lymphatic abnormalities. The male:female ratio is 2:1, and is more common on the right side than the left. Chyle can be distinguished from exudates by its pH (7.4–7.8), high lipid content and preponderance of lymphocytes; and from transudates by its high protein and lipid content.

Ciliary dyskinesia

See Immotile cilia syndrome

Citrullinemia

See Urea cycle disorders

Cleft lip and cleft palate

Cleft lip may be an isolated condition or associated with cleft palate. It occurs in one in about 1.4 per 1000 live births. It is usually on the left side. Bilateral cleft lip can occur. It can vary from a slight notch to complete cleft into the floor of the nasal cavity. The rare median cleft lip is different genetically from the usual forms and may have its own specific syndromal associations, such as Ellis–van Creveld syndrome.

Isolated cleft palate occurs in about 1 in 2500 live births and is less common than cleft lip with cleft palate; the occurrence in other members of the family greatly increases the risk. In 8% of cases it is associated with multiple malformation syndromes. There is an X-linked form which is associated with ankyloglossia.

Cleft lip and palate can occur in a number of autosomal, autorecessive, X-linked, chromosomal and non-mendelian conditions.

Cleidocranial dysplasia (dysostosis)

Cleidocranial dysplasia is an autosomal dominant condition characterized by multiple skeletal defects. The condition is familial in two-thirds of cases. The clavicles may be completely absent (the shoulders then being approximated in the midline) or have hypoplasia of the lateral end. The ribs can be short and the thorax small. The skull at birth may have very large fontanels, with the sutures closing late. The pelvic outlet may be very small in women, and Cesarean section may be required in childbirth. Dental dysplasias are common.

Cloacal exstrophy (dystrophy)

Other name Vesicointestinal fissure

Cloacal exstrophy is due to a failure of development of the urorectal septum and bladder exstrophy. The incidence is 1 in 250 000 live births. It is characterized by a large defect of the lower abdominal wall, bladder exstrophy, intestinal protrusion, an exposed strip of cecum, which represents the hindgut, small hemibladders and small hemiphalluses.

Clouston syndrome

Clouston syndrome is an autosomal dominant condition characterized by dystrophic nails, thick dyskeratotic palms and soles, hyperpigmented patches on the skin, strabismus, and sometimes cataracts and mental retardation.

Cloverleaf skull deformity syndrome

Cloverleaf skull deformity syndrome is characterized by a trilobed skull, exophthalmos, downward displacement of the eyes, a beaked nose and projecting jaws. It is due to an intrauterine synostosis of the coronal and lamboid sutures. Other skeletal abnormalities may be present.

Coffin-Lowry syndrome
See Coffin–Siris syndrome

Coffin-Siris syndrome

Other name Coffin–Lowry syndrome

Coffin–Siris syndrome is a congenital syndrome of multiple abnormalities, including an abnormal facies with thick eyebrows, a flat nasal bridge and anteverted lip, excess hair on the trunk and limbs, decrease of scalp hair, absence of the fifth fingernails and toenails and, sometimes, absence of the fifth fingers, dislocation of the head of the radius, small patellae, congenital heart defects, inguinal hernia, hypotonia, and mental retardation. Males can show the full syndrome; females may show only abnormal digits and mental retardation. Respiratory infections are common.

COFS syndrome
See Cerebro–oculo–facio–skeletal syndrome

Cohen syndrome

Cohen syndrome is characterized by microcephaly, maxillary hypoplasia, large ears, chorioretinal dystrophy, narrow hands and feet, slim fingers, lordosis, cryptorchidism, mental retardation, and delayed puberty. Obesity is likely in mid-childhood.

Collodion baby

Collodion baby is one born encased in a shiny membrane, the baby looking as if varnished all over. After a few days, the membrane starts to crack and peel off, leaving the skin beneath normal or bright red, and sometimes forming new membrane. The internal organs are normal. Complications include temperature instability, dehydration, pneumonia, and skin infections.

Coloboma

Coloboma is a notch or gap in the iris of the eye due to arrest of normal embryonic fissure closure at 4–6 weeks' gestation. It can be transmitted as an autosomal dominant trait and can be associated with a multiple system disorder. It is usually located inferiorly and rarely disturbs vision.

Colonic atresia

Atresia of the colon can occur in any part of the colon but is most common in the ascending colon. The colon may be much reduced in length and there may be other congenital abnormalities of the gastro-intestinal tract. Clinical features are vomiting, abdominal distension, and a failure to pass meconium.

Color blindness

Color blindness is inherited as an X-linked recessive disorder. It occurs in 8% of men and less than 0.5% of women. It occurs in many forms. The commonest form is red–green blindness, partial or complete, in which the individual has difficulty in distinguishing green from red. Other deficiencies include inability to distinguish clearly reds, greens, blues, and violets, and a total color blindness. Many individuals are unaware of their color blindness. The rare total color blindness (monochromatism) is autosomal recessive, except for the even rarer 'blue cone' type, which is X-linked.

Colpocephaly

Colpocephaly is a congenital abnormality of the brain in which the fetal configuration of the cerebral ventricles persists into postnatal life, with the occipital horns being greatly dilated. Clinical features can be tetraparesis, choreoathetosis and optic atrophy.

Complete heart block

Congenital complete heart block occurs in 1 in 20000 live births. Eighty per cent are in the children of women with systemic lupus erythematosus or other autoimmune diseases.

Complete transposition of the great arteries

In complete transposition of the great arteries the aorta arises anteriorly from the right ventricle and the pulmonary artery posteriorly from the left ventricle, with systemic blood passing through the right heart chambers into the body and pulmonary venous blood passing through the left heart chambers and returning to the lungs. The incidence is 1 in 4500 live births and the male:female ratio is 2:1. The presenting clinical feature is cyanosis. The infant's survival depends upon mixing between the two circuits. It may be an isolated abnormality or associated with atresia or stenosis of the pulmonary valve, defects of the atrial or ventricular septa, and abnormalities of the atrioventricular valves.

Congenital rubella syndrome

Congenital rubella syndrome is a malformation complex involving a fetus infected *in utero* by a mother with active rubella (German measles) in the early months of pregnancy. The malformations can include patent ductus arteriosus, pulmonary valve stenosis, ventricular septal defect, cataracts, deafness, microcephaly, enlarged liver and spleen, interstitial pneumonia, and mental retardation.

Contractural arachnodactyly
See Beals syndrome

Conradi syndrome

Other name Conradi–Hünermann syndrome

Conradi syndrome is a familial (dominant) or sporadic syndrome characterized by short stature, chondrodystrophy with characteristic punctate calcification of the epiphyses (visible on X-ray) and scaling of the skin, which clears up during the first year of life and leaves behind atrophic areas and areas of cicatricial alopecia. Renal disease, congenital heart disease and mental retardation can be present.

Conradi–Hünermann syndrome
See Conradi syndrome

Cornelia de Lange syndrome

Other name De Lange syndrome; Brachmann–de Lange syndrome

Cornelia de Lange syndrome is an autosomal recessive inherited disorder characterized by a 'lobster-claw' deformity of the hands, short stature, microcephaly, cleft lip and palate, optic atrophy, upturned nose, bushy eyebrows, hirsutism, low hair-line, beaked upper lip and notched lower lip, marbled skin, webbed toes, hypoplastic nipples, failure to thrive, and mental retardation. Chromosomal abnormalites, including ring chromosome 3, are present in some patients.

Corpus callosum agenesis

Absence of the corpus callosum may be partial or complete. Most cases are isolated; in some families, it occurs as an X-linked recessive condition. It occurs in a number of metabolic diseases and syndromes of the nervous system.

Cortical dysplasia

Cortical dysplasia is a localized disturbance of the cerebral cortex in which there are giant astrocytes and neurons and chaotic organization. It can be recognized by magnetic resonance imaging. It is a cause of partial epilepsy.

Cor triatriatum

Cor triatriatum is a heart with three atrial chambers, the pulmonary veins emptying into an accessory chamber above the left atrium and communicating with it by a small opening. It is due to a failure of resorption of the common pulmonary vein with partitioning of the left atrium into a proximal channel, which receives the pulmonary venous return, and a distal channel, which is continuous with the mitral valve. There is an obstruction to the ventricular inflow by an obstruction to the pulmonary venous return.

See also Heart malformations

Cranio-carpo-tarsal syndrome
See Freeman–Sheldon syndrome

Cranio-cerebello-cardiac dysplasia
See C3 syndrome

Craniofacial dysostosis
See Crouzon syndrome

Cranio-fronto-nasal dysplasia

Cranio-fronto-nasal dysplasia is characterized by synostosis of the coronal suture, frontonasal dysplasia (hypertelorism, widow's peak, bifid tip of the nose), cutaneous syndactyly, broad thumbs, grooved nails, sloping shoulders, and scoliosis.

Craniometaphyseal dysplasia

Craniometaphyseal dysplasia can occur as an autosomal dominant, and more severely as an autosomal recessive condition. It is characterized by hyperostosis of the skull, facial bones and mandible, with compression of the brain and cranial nerves.

Craniosynostosis

Craniosynostosis is premature fusion of one or more cranial sutures. It can occur as a single anomaly or as part of a multiple malformation syndrome. Premature fusion of the sagittal suture causes scaphocephaly – a long narrow skull with a prominent forehead and occipit. Premature fusion of one coronal suture causes brachycephaly – a short wide skull. Premature fusion of both coronal sutures causes plagiocephaly – an asymmetric skull with flattening of one half of the forehead and flattening of the contralateral occiput. *Kleeblattschadel* is a cloverleaf configuration of the skull due to fusion of multiple sutures. Synostosis of the sagittal sinus is the commonest type; about 2% are familial. Synostosis of the coronal sutures is the next most common type; about 8% are familial. Mental retardation is a common feature, and the more sutures are involved, the more likely it is to occur. Craniosynostosis is a feature of many congenital syndromes.

Craniosynostosis-radial aplasia syndrome
See Baller–Gerold syndrome

Cranium bifidum

Cranium bifidum is a failure of fusion of the posterior mid-line of the skull.

See also Encephalocele

Cretinism

Cretinism is due to severe maternal iodine deficiency during the first half of pregnancy. The affected child is likely to show severe mental retardation, spastic diplegia, deafness, strabismus, nystagmus, and, sometimes, goiter.

Cri-du-chat syndrome

Cri-du-chat syndrome is characterized by deformity of the larynx (a coarse unpleasant sound being produced), microcephaly, hypertelorism, prominent ears, short stature and severe mental retardation. There is loss of chromosomal material from the distal portion of the short arm of chromosome 5.

Crome syndrome

Crome syndrome is an autosomal recessive disorder characterized by congenital cataracts, renal tubular necrosis, encephalopathy, small stature, epilepsy and mental retardation.

Cross syndrome

Cross syndrome is characterized by ocular hypopigmentation, cutaneous hypopigmentation, athetosis, spastic tetraplegia, and severe mental retardation.

Crouzon syndrome

Other name Craniofacial dysostosis

Crouzon syndrome is an autosomal dominant condition characterized by premature closure of the cranial sutures, an abnormally shaped head, hypertelorism, a beaked nose, and hypoplasia of the maxilla. The skull deformity may be a brachycephaly, scaphocephaly, trigonocephaly (triangular shape due to a mid-line angulation of the frontal bone), or cloverleaf. Other features can be strabismus, nystagmus, exophthalmos, a highly arched or cleft palate, malocclusion of the teeth, and increased intracranial pressure.

Cryptophthalmos syndrome

Other name Fraser syndrome

Cryptophthalmos syndrome is an autosomal recessive condition characterized by cryptophthalmos (a defect of the anterior part of the eye), absence of palpebral fissures, absence of eyelashes and eyebrows, partial cutaneous syndactyly, imperfect sexual development (male: cryptorchidism, hypospadias; female: bicornuate uterus, vaginal atresia), renal agenesis, and laryngeal atresia or stenosis.

Cryptorchidism

Cryptorchidism (maldescent of the testes) is a common congenital abnormality of males. The smaller the testis the greater is the incidence. It occurs in 30% of preterm infants, 3.4% of full-term infants, and 0.2% of adult men. Its cause is uncertain: the most likely cause is hormonal; short blood vessels, intra-abdominal adhesions, and maldevelopment of the cremasteric muscle have been blamed. The testis may be located within the abdomen, in the canal between the internal and external rings, and ectopically (in the perineum, femoral canal, superficial inguinal pouch, suprapubic area, or in the opposite scrotal compartment). Before puberty, the testis is histologically normal; after puberty, it remains small, with a thickened capsule, failure of germinal-cell elements, and absent or rare spermatogenesis. About 90% of men with undescended testes are infertile. Complications can be neoplasia (about 10% of testicular tumors develop in undescended testes), abnormalities of the epididymis and vas deferens, and cystic fibrosis.

Currarino syndrome

Currarino syndrome is a congenital disorder characterized by a triad of anorectal malformation, a sacral bony abnormality, and a presacral mass, which can be teratoma, a meningocele, a hamartoma or an enteric duplication. A rectospinal canal fistula may be present.

Cutis hyperplastica

See Ehlers–Danlos syndrome

Cutis laxa

Cutis laxa is a congenital disorder characterized by laxation of the skin which hangs in baggy folds. It can be an autorecessive and an autosomal dominant condition.

Cutis marmorata telangiectatica congenita

Cutis marmorata telangiectatica congenita is a vascular lesion usually involving the skin of the trunk and lower limbs. Thrombosis can occur and cause ulcerations, which heal, leaving a scar. It tends to improve with age.

Cyclopia

Cyclopia is a condition in which there is a single rudimentary eye. The incidence is about 1 in 1 000 000 births. The maternal age may be markedly increased. It is likely to be associated with multiple congenital abnormalities such as median defect of the face, holoprosencephaly, microcephaly, caudal defects of the spine, malformed or absent kidneys, pulmonary aplasia, and absence of external genitalia.

Cystathioninemia

Cystathioninemia is an autosomal recessive condition in which, due to deficency of cystathionase, there is increased cystathionine in blood and urine. Most children appear normal; hyperactivity and mental retardation have been seen in others. It occurs in two forms, one of which reponds to vitamin B6 (pyridoxine).

Cystic hygroma

Cystic hygroma is derived from lymphoid tissue and, developing in the lateral areas of the neck, can cause respiratory obstruction.

D

Dandy–Walker syndrome

Dandy–Walker syndrome is a hydrocephalus in a neonate, due to a failure of development of the foramina of Luschka and Magendie in the roof of the fourth ventricle of the brain. Because of this failure, the cerebrospinal fluid cannot pass into the subarachnoid space and in consequence accumulates in the ventricles.

Dead fetus syndrome

Dead fetus syndrome is characterized by death of the fetus and either its retention *in utero* or its delivery macerated, in association with a hemorrhagic syndrome, within three weeks of its apparent death. Hypofibrinogenemia occurs in about 25% of patients in whom a dead fetus is retained *in utero*. Fibrinogen-related antigens, possibly derived from the dead fetus, can be present in increasing amounts, with the production of disseminated intravascular coagulation. In twin pregnancy, one of the two fetuses sharing a placenta can die and the other survive, but with cerebral, renal or splenic necrosis.

Deaf mutism

Other name Severe congenital sensorineural deafness

The incidence is about 1 in 1000 births. About 40–50% of cases are autosomal, about 10% are autosomal dominant, and the rest are due to unknown or undetected environmental factors. The risk in sibs of an isolated case is about 1 in 10. When consanguinity exists, autosomal recessive inheritance is more likely, and the risk is about 1 in 4. Should a couple have a second affected child, autosomal inheritance is almost certain. The risk for offspring of healthy sibs is under 1% in the absence of consanguinity or of deafness in the family of the other partner. The risk for offspring of an affected individual who is an isolated case and married to a normal person is around 5%.

De Barsy syndrome

De Barsy syndrome is an autosomal recessive disorder characterized by cutis laxa, skin atrophy, corneal clouding, cataracts, microcephaly, large ears, joint hyperextensibility, and mental retardation.

Debré-de Toni-Fanconi syndrome

See Fanconi syndrome

de Lange syndrome

See Cornelia de Lange syndrome

Demarquay syndrome

Other name Lip pit syndrome

Demarquay syndrome is characterized by a familial pit on the lower lip and, sometimes, cleft palate.

De Sanctis-Cacchione syndrome

De Sanctis-Cacchione syndrome is a recessive inherited condition with degeneration of cerebral and cerebellar neurons. Clinical features include microcephaly, short stature, gonadal dysplasia, xeroderma pigmentosa, mental retardation, progressive neurological and mental deterioration with spasticity, choreoathetosis, ataxia, and shortening of the Achilles tendon.

Dextrocardia

Dextrocardia is the condition in which the heart is in the right side of the chest, either because it has been displaced from its normal left-sided position or because it is a mirror-image dextrocardia. Mirror-image dextrocardia is usually associated with complete situs inversus (the abdominal organs being in reversed positions, left and right); and other congenital heart anomalies are present. It can be an isolated dextrocardia with the abdominal organs being in the normal position (situs solitus); other congenital heart anomalies are very common.

Diaphragmatic eventration

Eventration of the diaphragm is due to deficiency of muscle development or to absence or paralysis of the phrenic nerves. The diaphragm wholly or partly is composed of fibrous tissue. Small areas of fibrosis might not produce clinical features. Generalized fibrosis results in an elevated dome of the diaphragm, minimal movements of the diaphragm, lung hypoplasia, and respiratory distress.

Diaphragmatic hernia

A congenital hernia of the diaphragm is due to a failure of fusion of the diaphragmatic leaflets during the 8–10th weeks of fetal life. The incidence is 1 in 4000 births. The defect is usually posterolateral at the foramen of Bochdalek or, rarely, anterolateral at the foramen of Morgagni. The defect may be large or small. The communication between peritoneal and pleural cavities enables abdominal organs to enter the chest, displace the mediastinum, and compress the developing lungs, which can become hypoplastic. The condition can be diagnosed radiologically antenatally, with visualization of the stomach in the chest as a bad prognostic sign. Clinical features are rapid and difficult respiration, cyanosis, a scaphoid abdomen, bowel sounds in the chest, and an apparent dextrocardia due to displacement of the mediastinum. Elevated pulmonary vascular resistance can cause persistence of the fetal circulation. The mortality is 30–50%, with death usually due to severe pulmonary hypoplasia.

Diastematomyelia

Diastematomyelia is a congenital condition in which the spinal cord is bisected by a cartilaginous or bony septum which extends from the back of a vertebral body in front to the dura or laminar arch behind, usually in the lower thoracic or lumbar region. Clinical features can be pes cavus, talipes varus, or atrophy of a lower limb. Disturbances of gait can appear when the child starts to walk. Over the site of the lesion, there can be a lipoma, a tuft of hair, or a hemangioma.

Diastrophic dysplasia

Diastrophic dysplasia is an autosomal recessive disorder with variable expression and is characterized by short stature, cervical kyphosis, thoracolumbar kyphoscoliosis, joint contractures, external ear abnormalities, and cleft palate (25% of cases). Other features can be deafness, stenosis of larynx and trachea, facial hemangioma, and lateral displacement of patellae.

DiGeorge syndrome

Other name Third and fourth pharyngeal pouch syndrome

DiGeorge syndrome is one of the contiguous gene syndromes. In it there is a small deletion from chromosome 22, detectable by gene mapping or the use of restriction fragment length polymorphism. The parathyroid glands are absent, the thymus is absent or aplastic and a cell deficiency occurs during the first 3 months of life. Clinical features include severe chronic infections (to which resistance is low), deformities of the ears, nose and mouth, abnormalities of the great vessels, obstruction of the aortic arch, hypoparathyroidism, tetany and cardiac failure.

Digito-reno-cerebral syndrome

See Eronen syndrome

Distal arthrogryposis syndrome

Distal arthrogryposis syndrome is an autosomal dominant condition characterized mainly by congenital contractures of the distal joints. The hand is tightly clenched with medially overlapping fingers and ulnar deviation. The feet may show calcaneovalgus, equinovarus or other deformities. The hips may be dislocated and the knees have flexion contractures. Other features can be hernias, cryptorchidism, and slight scoliosis.

Distichia syndrome

Distichia syndrome is an autosomal dominant disorder characterized by distichia (a double row of eyelashes on the lids with one or both rows turned inwards onto the eyeball), lymphedema of the legs developing in childhood or adolescence, and, sometimes, vertebral defects and epidural cysts.

Donohue syndrome

Other name Leprechaunism

Donohue syndrome is an autosomal recessive disoder characterized by a broad nose, hypertelorism, low-set large ears, short stature, bone dystrophy, large penis in males, ovarian cysts in females, sexual precocity, and mental retardation. It may be due to a failure of cellular response to insulin, with hyperinsulinemia, hyperglycemia, and hyperplasia of the islets of Langerhans.

(A leprechaun is an ugly but friendly little spirit who helps Irish housewives with their work.)

DOOR syndrome

DOOR syndrome includes:
D – deafness
O – onychodystrophy
O – osteodystrophy
R – retardation (mental)
It may be the same as Eronen syndrome.

Douane retraction syndrome

Douane retraction syndrome is a congenital disorder of eye movement thought to be due to a failure of cranial nerve III to innervate the cell bodies of the eye muscles and its replacement by abnormal innervation from cranial nerve VI. It has also been attributed to an abnormal development of the nucleus of cranial nerve VI. Clinical features are abduction deficiency, globe retraction, and palpebral fissure narrowing on attempted eye adduction. The lateral rectus muscle is usually fibrotic.

Down syndrome

Other name Trisomy 21 syndrome

The presence of three chromosomes number 21 causes severe mental retardation (IQ usually under 50) and characteristic physical abnormalities. The only known etiological factor is increased maternal age. The risk of Down syndrome in a baby per 1000 live births is 0.7 for a woman under 30 years of age; for a woman of 40–44 years it is 13.1 per 1000 live births, and for a woman over 45 it is 34.6 per 1000 live births. However, because young women have more babies than older women, most Down syndrome babies are born to young mothers – 51% to mothers under 30 years and 72% to mothers under 35 years.

Physical features include short stature, small round head, short neck, mongoloid slant of the eyes, epicanthic fold of the eyelids, enlarged fissured tongue, transverse palmar crease, muscle hypotonia, rough skin, and obesity in older patients. Congenital heart disease occurs in about 50% of patients and is a major cause of morbidity and mortality; the defects can be endocardial cushion defect, septal defect, Fallot tetralogy, and patent ductus arteriosus. Gastrointestinal abnormalities include pyloric stenosis, duodenal atresia or stenosis, and Hirschsprung disease. Pulmonary infection is common. Tonsillar hypertrophy can cause obstructive sleep apnea. There may be defects of the cervical spine; atlantoaxial subluxation can cause a stiff neck, or be fatal. Some patients have alopecia areata. There is an increased incidence of acute lymphoblastic leukemia. Over the age of 30 years, there is a high incidence of orofacial dyskinesia. In the fourth and fifth decades, the pathological changes of Alzheimer disease can develop in the brain.

Some patients can show mosaicism – a mixture of normal and trisomic cells – and in these the IQ can be in the 70s, and the physical abnormalities may not be so marked.

The condition can be diagnosed *in utero* by chorion villus biopsy at 11 weeks (which carries a risk of abortion of 2–3%) or amniocentesis at 16 weeks (which carries a risk of abortion of 1–2%). Tests of maternal blood are for raised activity level of urea-resistant neutrophil alkaline phosphatase and a 'triple marker test' of estriol, human chorionic gonadotropin, and α-fetoprotein.

Dubowitz syndrome

Dubowitz syndrome is an autosomal recessive condition characterized by low birth weight, short stature, high sloping forehead, broad nasal bridge, short palpebral fissures, prominent dysplastic ears, sparse hair, eczema and, sometimes, mental retardation.

Duodenal atresia

Atresia of the duodenum is a complete obstruction between stomach and duodenum, probably due to a failure of recanalization during the 8–10th weeks of fetal life. There can be a complete separation of stomach and duodenum, the two may be connected by a fibrous band, or there may be an obstruction with continuity of bowel wall. There may be a maternal history of hydramnios. The clinical feature is vomiting. Associated conditions can be multiple atresias of the bowel, esophageal atresia, annular pancreas, and cardiovascular malformations. It can be a feature of Down syndrome.

Duodenal stenosis

Stenosis of the duodenum can be due to an intrinsic defect of the duodenal wall or to pressure on it by an aberrant superior mesenteric artery, a preduodenal vein, a peritoneal band, or an annular pancreas. The clinical feature is vomiting, which is likely to be bile-stained, as the stenosis is usually beyond the opening of the bile duct.

Dyggve–Melchior–Clausen syndrome

Dyggve–Melchior–Clausen syndrome is an autosomal recessive condition characterized by coarse facies, large jaws, microcephaly, short trunk, dwarfism, barrel chest, clawing of the fingers, subluxation of the hips, malalignment of the spine, and mental retardation. X-rays show dysplasia of the epiphyses and metaphyses of the proximal limb bones.

Dyscephalia mandibulo-oculofacialis
See Hallermann–Streiff syndrome

Dyschondrosteosis
See Leri–Weill syndrome

Dyskeratosis congenita
See Zinsser–Engmann syndrome

Dysplasia epiphysealis multiplex

Dysplasia epiphysealis multiplex is an autosomal dominant condition with a wide variation of expression. It is characterized by small irregular epiphyses, shortness of stature, short metacarpals and phalanges, slow growth and, later, waddling gait and osteoarthritis.

Dysplastic extremity-polydactyly-dyscrania syndrome

Dysplastic extremity–polydactyly–dyscrania syndrome is of uncertain etiology. It is characterized by unilateral tibial defect, polydactyly, macrotrigonocephaly, short and imperfectly developed limbs, and a liability to dislocations of the hips and knees.

E

Eagle–Barrett syndrome
See Prune belly syndrome

Early amnion rupture syndrome

Early amnion rupture syndrome is due to rupture of the amnion in early embryogenesis. Digits and extremities can be trapped in residual bands of amnion and can show deep circumferential constriction rings, or become amputated. The abnormalities are usually asymmetric. Structures proximal to a band are normal; structures distal to it are swollen as a result of obstruction to venous and lymphatic returns. Other features can be hemorrhage and necrosis of craniofacial structures and of the trunk.

See also Limb-body wall syndrome

Ebstein tricuspid valve anomaly

Ebstein tricuspid valve anomaly is a downward displacement of the leaflets of the tricuspid valve, and thinning of the atrialized right ventricle, which becomes dilated. Cyanosis is a feature if the foramen ovale is patent.

See also Heart malformations

Ectodermal dysplasia clefting syndrome
See EEC syndrome

Ectopia cordis

Ectopia cordis is a protrusion of the heart and attached vessels through the aperture produced by a failure of the two halves of the sternum to unite. Gross congenital abnormalities of the protruded heart may be present.

Ectrodactyly

Other names Split hand; 'lobster claw' defect.

Ectrodactyly, as an isolated bilateral condition, is usually autosomal dominant; it can be autosomal recessive. Conditions in which it occurs include EEC syndrome.

EEC syndrome

Other names Ectrodactyly; ectodermal dysplasia clefting syndrome

EEC is an autosomal dominant condition characterized by:
E – ectrodactyly (split deformity of the hand and foot)
E – ectodermal dysplasia (anomalies of the teeth, hair, nails, sweat
    glands, and nasolacrimal ducts)
C – cleft lip and palate
Ectrodactyly may not always be present. The critical chromosomal region is 7q11.2–q21.3.

Ehlers–Danlos syndrome

Other name Cutis hyperplastica

Ehlers–Danlos syndrome is an inherited form of collagen abnormality of which 11 different variants have been described. It can be inherited as an autosomal dominant, an autosomal recessive, or an X-linked recessive condition. It is characterized by hyperelasticity of the skin, which is loose and thickened, hyperextensibility and subluxation of joints, due to loose capsules, and impaired wound healing, with the development of coarse scars. Angioid streaks are present in the fundi of the eyes, and retinal hemorrhages can occur. The skin, veins and tracheal mucosa are fragile. Bleeding can occur from the gastrointestinal tract, and the urinary tract, and from the skin after minor injury. Spontaneous pneumothorax can occur. Collagen in arterial walls can be affected, and aneurysms can occur and rupture spontaneously. Hypertension can be present, and the pulses in the extremities can be absent or weak, because of the hyperelasticity of arteries. Other features can be pseudoxanthoma elasticum, subcutaneous calcification after trauma, and infarction of the stomach.

Eisenmenger syndrome

Eisenmenger syndrome is any cardiac left-to-right shunt with pulmonary hypertension.

Ellis–van Creveld syndrome

Other name Chondroectodermal dysplasia

Ellis–van Creveld syndrome is an autosomal recessive disorder characterized by short limbs, a long narrow thorax, polydactyly, hypoplastic nails and teeth, and congenital heart defects such as atrial and ventricular defects and cleft mitral valve. Erupted teeth can be present at birth. Respiratory distress can occur, due to deficiency of tracheal and bronchial cartilage.

EMG syndrome

EMG syndrome is a congenital condition characterized by:
E – exomphalos
M– macroglossia
G – gigantism
Hypoglycemia can occur in the early days of life.

Encephalocele

Encephalocele is a herniation of brain tissue or meninges or both, through a defect in the skull. About 60% occur in the occipital region and the rest usually in the frontonasal region and, much less commonly, in other regions. An occipital encephalocele presents as a soft round mass in the midline and can vary in size. Microcephaly may be present and other associated conditions are midline facial cleft, meningomyelocele, and congenital heart disease. A frontonasal encephalocele presents as a round mass at the base of the nose.

Encephalomucocutaneous lipomatosis

Encephalomucocutaneous lipomatosis is of unknown etiology. It is characterized by macrocephaly, intracranial lipomatosis, soft tissue tumors of head and face, alopecia, porencephalic cysts, focal fits, and cerebral hemiatrophy.

Enchondromatosis
See Ollier syndrome

Endomyocardial abnormality

Endomyocardial abnormality is characterized by endocardial fibroelastosis, affecting mainly the left side of the heart, and hypertrophy of the left ventricular wall, with the chamber being either dilated or small. Death in infancy is likely.

See also Heart malformations

Epidermal nevus syndrome
See Fuerstein–Mimms syndrome

Epidermolytic hyperkeratosis
See Bullous ichthyosiform erythroderma

Epididymis

Congenital abnormalities of the epididymis are rare. They can be:

(1) Absence: can be associated with absence of the testis;

(2) Duplication: usually associated with polyorchidism;

(3) Abnormal descent or position: associated with abnormal descent of the testis; the epididymis can come to lie in front of the testis;

(4) Fusion abnormalities: there can be an absence of fusion between the ducts and the seminiferous tubules;

(5) Cystic dilatation.

The abnormalities have sometimes been attributed to the mother's exposure to diethylstilbestrol during pregnancy.

Epiloia
See Tuberous sclerosis

Epimerase deficiency
See Uridine diphosphate galactose-4-epimerase deficiency

Epispadias

Epispadias is a congenital deformity of the urethra, which, in men, opens on the dorsum of the penis or on the glans penis. In its most severe form, the condition is associated with exstrophy of the bladder. The incidence is 1 in 100 000 live births. The male:female ratio is 3:1. In males, the glans penis or the penis is split on its dorsal surface, with exposure of the urethra as a deep groove, which in severe cases can extend to the neck of the bladder. In females, the upper wall of the urethra is cleft.

Epulis

Congenital epulis is a benign tumor composed of vascular connective tissue, spindle-shaped cells and polyhedral or round cells covered by squamous epithelium. It arises from tissue overlying the bone of the upper or lower jaw. It projects into the mouth and interferes with swallowing.

Eronen syndrome

Other name Digito-reno-cerebral syndrome

Eronen syndrome is an autosomal recessive condition characterized by absence of the distal phalanges of the toes and fingers, renal defects and cerebral anomalies. It may be the same as DOOR syndrome.

Escobar syndrome

Escobar syndrome is an autosomal recessive condition characterized by webs of the neck, axillae, antecubital fossa, popliteal fossa, and intercrural areas, ptosis, micrognathia, cleft palate, syndactyly, permanent flexion of the fingers, equinovarus, cryptorchidism, and absence of labia majora.

Esophageal achalasia

Esophageal achalasia is a motility disorder of the esophagus in which there is inadequate peristalsis in the body of the esophagus and increased pressure in the lower esophageal sphincter and a failure of it to relax. Clinical features are vomiting and aspiration pneumonia.

Esophageal shortening

Other names Partial thoracic stomach; hiatus hernia

Congenital shortening of the esophagus is a condition in which there is a failure of the esophagus to elongate to its normal length, with a failure of the stomach to migrate caudally, or an abnormal development of the diaphragm. About 15-20% of the stomach is in the thorax. Clinical features are vomiting and aspiration pneumonia.

Esophageal stenosis

Congenital esophageal stenosis can be due to (1) a variety of esophageal atresia in which juxtaposed segments are separated by a thin diaphragm of mucous membrane or a full thickness of esophageal wall or (2) abnormal tissue (such as respiratory tissue) in the esophageal wall. Clinical features are vomiting and discomfort.

External auditory canal atresia

Congenital atresia of the external auditory canal can be of variable severity. There may be only a shallow pit, or no cavity at all. The atresia can be bilateral or unilateral. Associated conditions can be an abnormally small pinna and absence or anomalies of the middle or internal ear.

External ear disorders

Protruding ears

Other names Bat ear; lop ear

Protruding ears are a common condition due to an absence of the antihelical fold in the auricular cartilage.

Accessory auricles

Accessory auricles appear as small tags between the tragus and the angle of the mouth. They often contain cartilage.

Microtia

Microtia is abnormal smallness or absence of the external ear. Associated conditions can be cartilage abnormalities and partial or complete stenosis of the external auditory meatus. It can be a feature of trisomy 13–15 and trisomy 18.

Pre-auricular sinus

Pre-auricular sinus is a small blind pit present in front of the root of the helix. It can be bilateral or unilateral and can be familial.

Fabry syndrome

Other names Anderson–Fabry syndrome; angiokeratoma corporis diffusum

Fabry syndrome is an X-linked recessive disorder in which deficiency of the enzyme α-galactosidase causes the deposition of neutral glycosphingolipids in tissues and fluids. Clinical features occur in many systems.

(1) Peripheral neuropathy occurs with painful crises ('Fabry crises') of burning agonizing pain in the hands and feet, radiating elsewhere and lasting from minutes to days; the pain can increase in frequency and intensity with age. Between attacks, unpleasant paresthesiae are present in the hands and feet, and attacks of pain can occur in the abdomen and flanks.

(2) Dark-red to bluish-red purpura-like spots appear on the lower trunk, buttocks and thighs.

(3) Cardiac involvement is shown by anginal pain, myocardial ische-mia, mitral insufficiency, enlargement of the heart, and conges-tive heart failure. The electroencephalogram (EEG) shows abnormalities.

(4) Involvement of the cerebral arteries causes cerebral thromboses, cerebral hemorrhage, and cerebral degeneration, with the pro-duction of mental deterioration and personality changes.

(5) Involvement of the eyes can cause cataracts and vascular lesions of the conjunctiva and retina.

(6) Involvement of the kidneys interferes with renal function and leads to death in early adult life from chronic renal failure.

(7) Involvement of other organs can cause chronic bronchitis, deteri-oration of pulmonary function, lymphedema of the legs, diar-rhea, retarded growth and puberty, skeletal abnormalities, anemia, fatigue, and weakness.

Prenatal diagnosis can be made by assay of α-galactosidase-A activity in chorionic villi or cultured amniotic cells obtained by amniocentesis.

Facial hemiatrophy
See Parry–Romberg syndrome

Facio–digital–genital syndrome
See Aarskog syndrome

Fallot tetralogy syndrome

Fallot tetralogy syndrome is a congenital disorder of the heart consisting of a ventricular septal defect, narrowing of the right ventricular outflow or stenosis of the pulmonary artery, overriding or dextroposition of the aorta, and right ventricular hypertrophy. It accounts for about 10% of all forms of congenital heart disease. Clinical features are cyanosis from birth or developing in the first year of life, retarded growth, dyspnea on exertion, clubbing of the fingers and toes, and polycythemia. A right ventricular impulse and thrill may be felt along the left border of the sternum. On auscultation, the second heart sound is single and the pulmonary component rarely heard; a mid-systolic murmur is usually present over the base of the heart.

See also Heart malformations

Falls–Kertsz syndrome

Falls–Kertsz syndrome involves congenital distichiases (secondary rows of eyelashes) and chronic lymphedema of the lower extremities.

Familial atypical multiple-mole–melanoma syndrome

Familial atypical multiple-mole–melanoma syndrome is an autosomal dominant inherited condition in which there is a variable predisposition to cutaneous malignant melanoma. It is characterized by the recognition of a family whose members have the cutaneous phenotypes of multiple atypical nevi, a total or multiple-mole count per person greater than the normal, and single or multiple melanomas. Cell cultures from melanocytes from atypical nevi and fibroblasts from normal skin of affected members of the family show an increased frequency of cells with non-random chromosomal rearrangements (translocation, deletions, inversions).

Familial neurovisceral lipoidosis
See Generalized gangliosidosis syndrome

Fanconi syndrome

Other names Renal tubular acidosis; Debré–de Toni–Fanconi syndrome

Fanconi syndrome is an autosomal recessive condition characterized by short stature, microcephaly, mental retardation, abnormalities of the radius, a reduced number of carpal bones, hypoplasia or aplasia of the thumb, absent radial pulse, hypoplastic bone marrow, congenital disease of the heart, hyperpigmentation of the skin, weakness, congenital dislocation of the hip, renal malformations, and gradual liver failure, with death likely before the age of 10 years. There is a disorder of the proximal renal tubules, with a defect in the reabsorption of glucose, amino acids, phosphate and potassium. Loss of calcium and phosphate causes hypoglycemia and hypophosphatemia. Calcium is withdrawn from bone, causing renal rickets. Nephrocalcinosis can occur.

Faucial pillar abnormalities

Faucial pillar abnormalities can be congenital perforation of one or both palatoglossal folds, or congenital absence of a palatoglossal fold associated with absence of the tonsil on the same side.

Femoral hypoplasia–unusual facies syndrome

Femoral hypoplasia–unusual facies is a very rare condition characterized by hypoplasia or absence of femur and fibula, hypoplasia of the humerus, restricted movement of the elbow, and unusual facies, with short nose, hypoplasia of alae, micrognathia, cleft palate, abnormalities of the vertebral column, absent or dysplastic kidney, and cryptorchidism. Maternal diabetes mellitus can be an association.

Fetal akinesia/hypokinesia sequence
See Pena–Shokeir syndrome

Fetal alcohol syndrome

Fetal alcohol syndrome is due to excessive drinking of alcohol by a pregnant woman. The child may show fetal growth retardation, cardiac defects (especially septal defects and Fallot tetralogy), maxillary hypoplasia, prominent lower jaw and forehead, small palpebral fissures, small eyes, unilateral ptosis, growth retardation, mental retardation, and abnormal neurobehavioral development.

Fetal face syndrome

See Robinow syndrome

Fetal phenytoin (hydantoin) syndrome

Fetal phenytoin (hydantoin) syndrome is due to an epileptic mother taking this drug during pregnancy. Fetal features can be growth deficiency, wide anterior fontanel, hypertelorism, depressed nasal bridge, cleft lip and palate, hypoplasia of distal phalanges, short neck, umbilical and inguinal hernia, rib abnormalities, and strabismus. Other features can be pulmonary valvular stenosis, aortic valvular stenosis, patent ductus arteriosus, coarctation of the aorta, microcephaly, ambiguous genitalia, and undescended testes.

Fetal rubella syndrome

Maternal rubella can cause serious fetal defects, especially if the mother is infected during the first 12 weeks of pregnancy. The usual features are low birth weight, congenital heart disease (pulmonary stenosis, patent ductus arteriosus), microcephaly, deafness, and eye defects (microphthalmia, cataracts, glaucoma). Other features can be an enlarged liver, jaundice, an enlarged spleen, purpura, thrombocytopenia, myocarditis and encephalitis.

A 'late-onset' rubella syndrome can occur. The affected infant shows minimal signs at birth, but at the age of 3–6 months, develops a multisystem disorder with diarrhea, skin rash, pneumonia, and hypogammaglobulinemia with circulating immune complexes. Later complications can be diabetes mellitus, fits, and hypotonia.

Fetal smoking syndrome

Smoking by a pregnant woman can cause intrauterine growth retardation, fetal hypoxia, placental abruption, miscarriage, premature rupture of membranes in labor, premature delivery, low Apgar scores (a method of assessing and recording a neonate's skin color, muscle tone, respiratory effort, heart rate, and responses to stimuli at 1, 5, and 10 min after birth), which can be associated with perinatal mortality, respiratory infections, and an increased risk of sudden infant death syndrome.

Fetal sodium valproate syndrome

Fetal sodium valproate syndrome is due to an epileptic woman taking this drug during pregnancy. Clinical features can be meningomyelocele, hypoplastic left heart, aortic valve stenosis, pulmonary atresia, cleft lip, short nose, epicanthal folds, and mental retardation.

Fetal tretinoin (retinoic acid) syndrome

The taking of tretinoin (retinoic acid) immediately before or during pregnancy can produce, in the child, central nervous system abnormalities (hydrocephaly, microcephaly, cerebellar defects), triangular facies, cleft palate, hypertelorism, depressed nasal bridge, cardiovascular abnormalities (Fallot tetralogy, ventricular septal defect, double-outlet right ventricle, truncus arteriosus communis, hypoplasia of the aortic arch, transposition of the great vessels), and abnormalities of the thymus. The child can be stillborn or die in infancy.

Fetal varicella syndrome

Fetal varicella syndrome (fetal chickenpox syndrome) is due to varicella infection of a pregnant woman in the first 3 or 4 months of pregnancy. Clinical features are low birth weight, cicatricial skin changes, hyoplasia of limbs, chorioretinitis, cerebral cortical atrophy, fits, and mental retardation.

FFU syndrome

FFU syndrome is a condition of unknown etiology characterized by:
FF – femoral and fibular defects (unilateral)
U – ulnar contralateral defects

FG syndrome

FG syndrome is named after the first families in which it was reported. It is an X-linked condition characterized by mental retardation, congenital hypotonia, structural anal anomalies (such as anal stenosis, imperforate anus, or anteriorly placed anus), constipation, macrocephaly, and characteristic facies, with an open mouth, a tall, broad forehead, and 'cowlicks' of the hairline. Other features can be agenesis of the corpus callosum, congenital heart disease, pyloric stenosis, and craniosynostosis.

Fibrochondrogenesis

Fibrochondrogenesis is a very rare, autosomal recessive disorder in which there is fibrosis of growth plate cartilage. Clinical features include short stature, large anterior fontanel, flat nasal bridge, cleft palate, short neck, flattened vertebrae, small chest, short limbs and abnormalities of the fingers. The infant may be stillborn or die shortly after birth.

Fibrodysplasia ossificans progressiva

Fibrodysplasia ossificans progressiva is an autosomal dominant disorder characterized by short hallux, sometimes a short thumb, and fibrous dysplasia in fasciae, tendons and aponeuroses, with the development, usually in childhood but at any time between fetal life and 25 years, of ossification in fibrous tissue and muscle, in the neck, trunk and proximal parts of limbs.

Fibro-osteolytic dwarfism
See Winchester syndrome

First and second arch syndrome
See Pierre Robin syndrome

Focal dermal hypoplasia
See Goltz syndrome

Fragile X syndrome

Fragile X syndrome is the most common cause of inherited mental retardation. The frequency is about 1 in 1000 in males and 1 in 2000 in females. The degree of mental retardation is severe to mild in boys and moderate to mild in girls. The syndrome derives its name from the presence of a hypochromic, ragged-looking constriction site at the distal end of the long arm of the X chromosome (Xq27), due to a failure of normal chromatid condensation during mitosis. The defect is due to expansion in a specific DNA triplet repeat (CGG) in a gene whose function is unknown. The size of the expansion correlates with the degree of mental retardation. Other features are likely to be slight enlargement of the head, a long face, large protruding ears, high-arched palate, aortic dilatation, mitral valve prolapse, a soft velvety skin, speech and language disturbances, hyperactivity, problems with attention and concentration, and autistic features.

François syndrome
See Hallermann–Streiff syndrome

Fraser syndrome
See Cryptophthalmos syndrome

Freeman–Sheldon syndrome

Other names Whistling face syndrome; cranio–carpo–tarsal syndrome

Freeman–Sheldon syndrome is usually an autosomal dominant condition (an autosomal recessive inheritance has been reported) in which the central area of the face bulges as if the person were whistling, probably due to a defect of the facial musculature. The face is stiff and mask-like. The mouth is small and pursed. Other features can be ulnar deviation of the hands, flexion of the fingers, bilateral talipes equinovarus, inguinal hernia, and incomplete descent of the testes.

Frontal sinus abnormalities

The frontal sinuses may vary in size and symmetry; each may be represented by a small air cell, or be absent.

Frontoethmoidal meningoencephalocele

Frontoethmoidal meningoencephalocele is a congenital abnormality in which meninges and cerebral tissue are herniated through a defect in the anterior cranium between the frontal and ethmoidal bones. It presents as an enlarging nasal or paranasal subcutaneous mass. It is rare in the USA and Europe and not uncommon in Southeast Asia. It may be due to maternal ingestion of ochratoxin A, an aflatoxin present in food in that part of the world, during hot humid months, and when stored for long periods in poorly ventilated rooms, and not destroyed by cooking.

Frontometaphyseal dysplasia

Frontometaphyseal dysplasia is an X-linked condition which affects males more severely than females. It is characterized by coarse facies, prominent supraorbital ridges, small mandible, teeth abnormalities, arachnodactyly, flexion defects of elbows, wrists, fingers, knees, and ankles, deafness, and wasting of muscles of the arms and legs, especially the hypothenar and interosseous muscles of the hands. Other features can be mental retardation, subglottic narrowing of the trachea, and obstructive uropathy.

Frontonasal dysplasia
See Median cleft-face syndrome

Fryns syndrome

Fryns syndrome is an autosomal recessive condition characterized by facial dysmorphism, cleft palate, cystic kidneys, diaphragmatic hernia, hypoplastic terminal phalanges and nails and abnormalities of the central nervous system and genitals. It is usually fatal.

Fucosidosis

Fucosidosis is an autosomal recessive condition of oligosaccharidosis, with Hurler-type facial dysmorphism, macrocephaly, thick eyebrows and hair, large tongue, short neck, claw hands, joint contractures, hepatomegaly, and cardiomegaly. Infantile, juvenile and adult forms can occur.

Fuerstein–Mimms syndrome

Other names Linear nevus sebaceus syndrome; nevus sebaceus of Jadassohn epidermal nevus syndrome; Soloman syndrome

Fuerstein–Mimms syndrome is characterized by a non-dermatomal linear pigmented nevus of the skin, skin defects of various kinds, eyelid colobomas, anomalies of the optic discs, skeletal abnormalities, and severe mental retardation. Other features can be corneal opacities, enlarged cerebral ventricles with cortical atrophy, and hypoplastic teeth.

G

G syndrome

See Opitz–Frias syndrome

Galactokinase deficiency

Galactokinase deficiency can occur in neonates as well as in older children. Galactose is present in large amounts in blood and urine and galactokinase activity in red cells is reduced or absent. The condition is usually asymptomatic in the neonatal state, but cataracts can develop later.

Galactosemia

Galactosemia is a genetic disorder transmitted as an autosomal recessive trait. Clinical features are likely to be present in the first few days of life and are jaundice, enlargement of the liver, poor feeding, lethargy, vomiting, and weight loss. Untreated, the child is likely to develop an *Escherichia coli* infection and meningitis. Untreated survivors are likely to develop cirrhosis of the liver, cataracts, and mental retardation. Treatment consists of eliminating from the diet all foods containing lactose, and, if this is started early in neonatal life, the prognosis for normal physical and mental development is good.

Gallbladder abnormalities

The gallbladder may be hypoplastic or absent, or it may be unconnected to the bile ducts or duodenum.

Gardner syndrome

Gardner syndrome is an autosomal dominant inherited disorder characterized by polyposis coli, bone tumors, epidermoid cysts, desmoid tumors, odontomes, and unerupted teeth. Malignant changes develop in the intestinal polyps in about one-third of cases.

Gastric antral diaphragm

A diaphragm or web of excessive endodermal tissue can block (usually incompletely) the antrum of the stomach. There may be an opening in the diaphragm through which food can pass. The clinical feature is non-bilious vomiting.

Gastric duplication

Gastric duplication is a doubling of the stomach by a tubular or spherical hollow organ with a mucosa similar to that of the stomach, small intestine or large intestine, lying alongside the greater curvature, and possibly communicating with the gastric lumen. Clinical features can be vomiting and a palpable abdominal mass. Associated features can be esophageal duplication and vertebral anomalies.

Gastric hypoplasia

Congenital hypoplasia of the stomach is the condition in which fetal rotation of the stomach does not occur, and the stomach remains in a primitive condition in which the fundus, body, antrum and pyloric canal do not develop. The clinical feature is vomiting. Associated conditions can be malrotation and esophageal fistula.

Gastric pyloric atresia

Gastric pyloric atresia is a complete obstruction of the pyloric canal due to a failure of canalization. There may be a history of maternal hydramnios. The clinical feature is vomiting.

Gastric pyloric stenosis

Pyloric stenosis is due to congenital hypertrophy of the pyloric muscle. The cause is unknown. The incidence is 1–3 in 1000 births. The male : female ratio is 4 : 1. Half the cases are firstborn children. There is a 7% incidence in siblings of affected parents. Clinical features are vomiting, which becomes projectile, visible gastric peristalsis, weight loss, dehydration, and a small, firm, palpable mass resembling an olive.

Gastroschisis

Gastroschisis is eventration of the abdominal contents due to a defect of the anterior abdominal wall. It is rarely associated with other congenital abnormalities. About 58% of affected infants are premature. Associated conditions are intestinal atresia and malrotation, and wound lesions.

Geleophysic dysplasia

Geleophysic dysplasia (*geleos physis* – happy nature (Greek)) is an autosomal recessive condition in which there is thought to be a defect of glycoprotein metabolism. It is characterized by a round face with a happy expression, short stature, short hands and feet, contractures of many joints, enlargement of the liver, and thickening of heart valves with valvular incompetence.

Genee-Wiedmann syndrome

Genee–Wiedmann syndrome is an autosomal recessive condition characterized by multiple congenital abnormalities, including acrofacial dysostosis, lower limb anomalies (absence of fibula, polydactyly, hypoplasia of the fifth toes), upper limb defects, supernumerary vertebrae, supernumerary nipples, congenital heart disease, and, sometimes, mental retardation.

Generalized gangliosidosis syndrome

Other names Familial neurovisceral lipoidosis; Caffey pseudo-Hurler syndrome

Generalized gangliosidosis syndrome is an autosomal recessive disorder in which there is a deficiency of the lysosomal enzyme β-galactosidase. It is characterized by prenatal and postnatal growth deficiency, coarse features, enlarged maxilla, macroglossia, claw hand, contractures at the elbows and knees, limitation of joint movement, hypoplastic vertebrae, enlarged liver, vacuolation of leukocytes and foam cells in the bone marrow, mental retardation and later spasticity, and, in about half the patients, a cherry-red spot in the macula of the eye.

Gershoni-Baruch-Machoul-Weiss-Blazer syndrome

Gershoni–Baruch–Machoul–Weiss–Blazer syndrome is a congenital disorder characterized by bilateral radioulnar synostosis, absence of the left thumb, three phalanges in the right thumb, umbilical hernia, diaphragmatic hernia, and a hepatic cyst.

Giant cell chondrodysplasia

Other name Atelosteogenesis

Giant cell chondrodysplasia is a condition in which multinucleated giant cells are scattered throughout resting cartilage. Clinical features are short stature, proximal shortness of limbs, absent fibula, flattened hypoplastic vertebrae, delayed ossification of proximal and middle phalanges, and, sometimes, cleft palate. All infants are still-born or die shortly after birth.

Gierke disease

See Glycogen storage disease I

Glossoptosis–apnea syndrome

Glossoptosis–apnea syndrome is characterized by pharyngeal obstruction due to prolapse of the tongue, which obstructs the airway, unilateral choanal atresia or stenosis, cyanosis, respiratory distress, and apneic episodes.

Glutaric aciduria I

Glutaric aciduria I is due to a defect in glutaric acid metabolism and is characterized by macrocephaly, bilateral atrophy of the temporal lobes, and, later in childhood, choreoathetosis, neurological deterioration, and mental retardation.

Glutaric aciduria II

Glutaric aciduria II is an autosomal recessive disorder in which there is increased glutaric acid in the urine. Clinical features are present on the first day of life and are characterized by metabolic acidosis, non-ketotic hypoglycemia, hypotonia, lethargy, and cardiomyopathy. Other features can be polycystic kidneys, omphalocele, and abnormalities of the external genitalia. Death in the neonatal period is common; survivors are likely to die in infancy.

Glycogen storage disease I

Other name Gierke disease

Glycogen storage disease I is a rare, autosomal recessive condition in which there is either a deficiency in glucose-6-phosphatase activity or a defect in the microsomal uptake of glucose-6-phosphate. There is an accumulation of glycogen in the liver and kidneys, and the neonate presents with an enlarged liver and sometimes hypoglycemia. Subsequently, the child can develop further enlargement of the liver, vomiting and severe hypoglycemic attacks.

Glycogen storage disease II

Other name Pompe syndrome

Glycogen storage disease II is characterized by failure to thrive, enlargement of the heart, enlargement of the tongue, and hypotonia.

Muscle biopsy shows normal structure with increased concentration of glycogen; leukocytes show an absence of α-glucosidase.

Glycogen storage disease III

Glycogen storage disease III is an autosomal recessive condition in which there is a deficiency of amylo-1,6-glucosidase. Clinical features are enlargement of the liver, growth retardation, and, sometimes enlargement of the spleen.

Goldenhar syndrome

Other name Ocular–auricular–vertebral dysplasia

Goldenhar syndrome is due to abnormalities of derivatives of first and second branchial arches. It is characterized by multiple ocular, skeletal and other abnormalities:

(1) Coloboma of the upper eyelids and iris, sub-conjunctival lipoma, epibulbar dermoid, cataracts, glaucoma and strabismus;

(2) Fusion of vertebrae, elongation of the odontoid process of the mandible, cleft of highly-arched palate; and

(3) Sensorineural deafness. Other features can be congenital heart disease (commonly Fallot's tetralogy and septal defects), renal abnormalities, and mental retardation.

Goltz syndrome

Other name Focal dermal hypoplasia

Goltz syndrome is a multisystem disorder. Of reported cases, 88% have been female. It is thought that an X-linked dominant inheritance with lethality in the male is the likely form of inheritance. Clinical features vary from slight to severe and vary in the organs involved. Cutaneous disorders occur in most cases. They are present at birth. They can be pink or red macules, from a few millimeters to several centimeters across, and are sometimes blistered or eroded (cutis aplasia), telangiectatic, pinkish or brown nodules, or raspberry-like papillomas on the face, ears, fingers, toes and perianal region. The hair is sparse and brittle, and there can be patches of alopecia. The nails can be absent or dystrophic. There can be skeletal deformities such as absence, hypoplasia or syndactyly of digits, lobster-like deformity of the hands, scoliosis, and asymmetry in size and shape of the face, trunk and limbs. Longitudinal striations (osteopathia striata) are visible in the shafts of long bones on X-ray. Other deformities can be spina bifida, dysplasia of the clavicle, dental abnormalities, horseshoe kidney, exomphalos and other hernias, strabismus, low-set ears, microcephaly, developmental delay and recurrent infections. Intelligence is usually normal, but mental retardation has been reported in 15% of cases.

Gonadal dysgenesis

See Turner syndrome

Gorlin syndrome

Other name Basal cell nevus syndrome

Gorlin syndrome is an autosomal dominant disorder characterized by frontoparietal bossing, broad nasal bridge, prognathism, misshapen teeth, ribs that are partially absent, fused or bifid, and scoliosis. The corpus callosum may be absent. In childhood, basal cell nevi develop on the face, neck, trunk and upper arms, and can become malignant. Other tumors may develop.

Grebe syndrome

Grebe syndrome is an autosomal condition of short distal parts of the limbs, in which the legs are more affected than the arms, the fingers resemble toes, and polydactyly may occur. The facies is normal. Many sufferers are stillborn or die in infancy.

Greig cephalopolysyndactyly syndrome

Greig cephalopolysyndactyly syndrome is an autosomal dominant condition characterized by macrocephaly, high forehead, frontal bossing, and polydactyly and syndactyly of the fingers and toes. Other features can be absence of the corpus callosum, slight hydrocephalus, and mental retardation.

Growth hormone deficiency

A rare form of growth hormone deficiency presents with hypoglycemia, jaundice, failure to thrive, and, in boys, microgenitalia. Most patients have multiple pituitary hormone deficiencies, especially deficiency of adrenocorticotropic hormone (ACTH) and thyroid stimulating hormone (TSH).

H

Hajdu–Cheney syndrome

Hajdu–Cheney syndrome is an autosomal dominant condition characterized by dysmorphic facies, broad thick eyebrows, maxillary and mandibular hypoplasia, persistent cranial fontanels and sutures, osteoporosis, and hyperextensibility of joints.

Hallermann–Streiff syndrome

Other names Dyscephalia mandibulo-oculofacialis; mandibulo-facial dyscephaly; François syndrome

Hallermann–Streiff syndrome is a syndrome of multiple congenital abnormalities, which can include malformations of the skull and facial bones, short stature, scoliosis, spina bifida, sensorineural deafness, beaked nose, hypoplastic nares, absent, brittle, extra or maloccluded teeth, diminished scalp- and body hair, sparse or absent eyebrows and eyelashes, microphthalmia, cataracts (which can absorb spontaneously), renal malformations, absence of radial bones and hypoplastic bone marrow. Progeria can develop in later life.

Hand–foot–genital syndrome

Hand–foot–genital syndrome is an association of mild malformations of the hands and feet with genital anomalies, including hypospadias in males and duplication of the genital tract in females.

Hand–heart syndrome
See Holt–Oram syndrome

Hanhart syndrome

Hanhart syndrome is a congenital condition characterized by absence or poor development of the tongue, small jaws, deformities of the limbs, and absence or poor development of the digits.

Happy puppet syndrome

Other name Angelman syndrome

Happy puppet syndrome is characterized by jerky movements, as if the child were being jerked by string like a puppet, severe mental retardation, an open-mouth expression, outbursts of laughter, absence of speech, maxillary hypoplasia, abnormal electroencephalogram (EEG), and poor physical development. Sixty percent have a small deletion of the long arm of chromosome 15 at 15q11–13, which is inherited from the mother.

HARD + E syndrome
See Walker–Warburg syndrome

Harlequin baby

Harlequin baby is a severe form of congenital ichthyosis, inherited as an autosomal recessive condition. The skin is discolored, hard, and cracked. Fissures develop in the neck, axillae and groin and over joints, which are fixed in flexion. Death from ventilation and feeding difficulties usually occurs within a few weeks of birth.

Hay–Wells syndrome
See AEC syndrome

Heart conduction defects

Congenital conduction defects of the heart are usually isolated cases. Familial forms occur in: Jervell–Lange–Nielsen syndrome (autosomal recessive); prolonged QT syndrome (autosomal dominant), with sudden death; children of mother with systemic lupus erythematosus (complete heart block); and late-onset heart block (dominant inheritance).

Heart malformations

Congenital heart malformations occur in at least 8–10 per 1000 births. With the exception of patent ductus arteriosus, the defect occurs within 6–8 weeks of fetal life. In 95%, the cause is unknown. Known causes are maternal rubella in the first 3 months, and certain chromosomal abnormalities, and the malformations occur in many congenital syndromes. Possible causes are maternal alcoholism or maternal taking of drugs. Cardiac malformations are found 10 times more often in stillborns than liveborns. Clinical features can be cyanosis of the lips and nail beds, abnormal pulsation in the suprasternal notch, chronic venous stasis, abnormal shape of the chest, abnormal heart sounds, puffiness of the eyelids, edema of the feet and pretibial and sacral areas, clubbing of the fingers, poor growth, and infections of the upper respiratory tract.

See also specific heart malformations

Heart valvular regurgitation

Congenital regurgitation of the aortic, pulmonary or mitral valve is present, with the murmurs and volume load on the relevant ventricle being characteristic for each lesion.

See also Heart malformations

Heart ventricular septal defects

Ventricular septal defects of the heart are the most common of cardiac abnormalities, with an incidence of about 1 per 1000 live births. It may be a single defect, or occur with other cardiac abnormalities. It may be no larger than a pin hole or so large that the ventricular septum is almost completely absent. A murmur may be the only sign, but, if the defect is large, congestive failure is likely to develop.

See also Heart malformations

Hecht syndrome

Other name Trismus pseudocamptodactyly syndrome

Hecht syndrome is an autosomal dominant condition with a male:female ratio of 1:2. It is characterized by short muscles and tendons in the arms and legs, flexion of fingers and toes, talipes equinovarus, and metatarsus adductus. There is limited opening of the mouth, which presents problems to anesthesiologists, dental surgeons, and surgeons operating on the mouth or throat.

Hemangiomas

Capillary and cavernous hemangiomas are benign tumors of blood vessels. They can be single or multiple. The incidence in neonates is about 1%, with a higher incidence in preterm infants. Hemangiomas may present as areas of pale, raised skin with some superficial dilated vessels. They tend to enlarge over the first 6 months and then, after a stationary period of some years, to resolve.

Hematogenous branchial cleft syndrome

Other name Branchio-oculofacial syndrome

Hematogenous branchial cleft syndrome is characterized by hemangiomatous branchial cysts, microphthalmos, myopia, coloboma, dysmorphic facies, and cleft lip and palate.

Hemifacial microsomia

Hemifacial microsomia is usually a sporadic condition. It is characterized by facial asymmetry, hypoplasia of the lower jaw, pre-auricular tags, and unilateral malformation of an ear.

Hemihypertrophy

Hemihypertrophy is the condition in which all or some of the structures on one side of the body are larger than those on the other side. Chromosomal abnormalities are sometimes present, and most cases are sporadic. Associated conditions can be adrenal cortical carcinoma, Wilms tumor, and hepatoblastoma, and tumors have been reported to occur in the opposite side. Hemihypertrophy is a feature of Beckwith–Wiedemann syndrome.

Hemoglobin Bart's hydrops syndrome

When there is deletion of all four genes on chromosome 16 coding for alpha globin chains, the only hemoglobin that can be synthesized in the second half of fetal life is Hb Bart's (Y4), which is not a good carrier of oxygen. The fetus is severely anemic and edematous and dies either late in pregnancy or shortly after birth. The mother has a high incidence of toxemia, obstructed labor, and post-partum hemorrhage.

Hereditary onycho-osteodysplasia

See Nail–patella syndrome

Hiatus hernia

See Esophageal shortening

Hidrotic ectodermal dysplasia

Hidrotic ectodermal dysplasia is an autosomal dominant condition characterized by hyperkeratosis of the palms and soles, absent, dystrophic or hypoplastic nails, and sparse hair. Sweating is normal. Teeth are small and liable to decay.

See also Hypohidrotic ectodermal dyplasia

Hippel–Lindau syndrome

Other name Lindau–Hippel syndrome

Hippel–Lindau syndrome is an autosomal dominant disorder characterized by angiomatous tumors of the retina, cutaneous nevi, hemangioblastoma of the cerebellum and spinal cord, a cerebellar syndrome, increased intracranial pressure, angiomatous or cystic lesions of the liver, pancreas, kidneys, lungs, epididymis and skin, pheochromocytoma, and renal cell carcinoma. A retinal angioma can cause hemorrhage into the eye, retinal detachment, and blindness. Neurofibromatosis (Recklinghausen syndrome) can be an associated condition. Hepatic and renal failure can occur; the prognosis is poor. Death can occur from these failures, an intracranial hemorrhage, or a cerebellar tumor.

HMC syndrome

Other name Bixler syndrome

HMC syndrome is characterized by:
H – hypertelorism
M – microtia (abnormal smallness of the pinna of the ear)
C – cleft lip or palate
Other features can be cardiac abnormalities, stenotic external auditory canals, and deafness.

Hoffman–Zurhelle syndrome

Other name Nevus lipomatides superficialis

Hoffman–Zurhelle syndrome is a developmental abnormality in which soft, fleshy nodules, usually present at birth, are present in the skin, usually on the lower part of the trunk.

Holocarboxylase synthetase deficiency

Holocarboxylase synthetase deficiency is due to a defect in this enzyme, which binds biotin to carboxylase. Clinical features are neonatal vomiting, lethargy, and signs of metabolic acidosis. Laboratory findings are acidosis, ketonuria, hyperammonemia and hypoglycemia.

Holoprosencephaly

Holoprosencephaly is a congenital abnormality of the brain, due to a failure of the telencephalon (primary cerebral vesicle) to divide and expand laterally. In some families, it is an autosomal recessive condition. In the severe form, there is a single large ventricular cavity within an undivided prosencephalic vesicle and a single median eye (cyclopia). In less severe forms, there are likely to be hypoplastic olfactory bulbs and tracts (arrhinencephaly) and facial abnormalities, such as cleft lip and palate, and hypertelorism. Less severely affected infants are likely to have attacks of apnea, fits, rigidity, and severe mental retardation.

Holt–Oram syndrome

Other name Hand–heart syndrome

In this autosomal dominant disorder, congenital cardiovascular malformations (commonly an atrial septal defect) are associated with an upper limb defect (commonly of the radius or thumb) in one person or separately in different members of a family. The syndrome is divided into two types: the complete type has both cardiovascular and upper limb deformities; the incomplete type has either the cardiovascular or the upper limb deformities.

Homocystinuria

Homocystinuria is an autosomal recessive condition in which there is a deficiency of cystathionine β-synthase, an enzyme which converts homocystine into cystathionine. The incidence is about 1 in 200 000 infants. The blood level of methionine is raised, and homocystine is present in small amounts in blood and urine. The neonate is usually normal; untreated, the child can develop ectopia lentis (dislocation of the lens of the eye), osteoporosis, and thromboembolism.

Horseshoe kidney

Horseshoe kidney is a fusion of the lower poles of the kidneys and probably develops during the 5–6th weeks of embryonic life. The fusion can arrest renal ascent at the level of the inferior mesenteric artery; the ureters may arise anteriorly due to prevention of rotation of the kidneys. It occurs about 1 in 400 live births, and is more common in males than in females. The condition usually remains asymptomatic throughout life. Complications can be infection, calculi, and hydronephrosis. Associated conditions can be obstruction at the pelvic–ureteric junction, hydronephrosis, undescended testes, hypospadias, bicornuate uterus, spina bifida, trisomy 18, oro–facio–digital syndrome, and Turner syndrome.

Howard-Young syndrome

Howard-Young syndrome is a congenital disorder characterized by microcephaly, polydactyly, cleft palate and lip, and developmental delay.

Hunter syndrome

Other name Mucopolysaccharidosis II

In this recessive sex-linked disorder there is a deficiency of iduronate sulfatase and an abnormal deposit of mucopolysaccharides in various tissues. An affected child may appear normal up to about 1 year of life. Clinical features include short stature, coarse facies, an enlarged liver and spleen, stiff joints, thoracoskeletal deformities which cause respiratory failure, laryngeal and pharyngeal obstruction, cardiac infiltration and failure, mental retardation and behavior problems. Other features can be ivory-colored nodules in the skin, progressive loss of sight and hearing, hydrocephalus, and degeneration of the functioning of the central nervous system. It is usually less severe than Hurler syndrome. Many patients die in childhood, but those with a minor form of the disorder can survive to early adult life. The condition can be diagnosed *in utero* by an assay of iduronate sulfatase in fetal blood.

Hurler syndrome

Other name Mucopolysaccharidosis I

Hurler syndrome is an autosomal recessive disorder in which there is a deficiency of α-L-iduronidase and an abnormal deposit of mucopolysaccharides in many tissues, especially in the brain, cornea, liver, spleen, and bone. An affected child may appear normal up to about 1 year of life, and then the head may be noticed to be becoming abnormally large. Clinical features are likely to include a large and abnormally shaped head, a short, thick neck, growth retardation, coarse facies, large tongue, hyperplastic gums, abnormally shaped and widely spaced teeth, corneal opacities, glaucoma, sensorineural deafness, an enlarged liver and spleen, a protuberant abdomen, umbilical and inguinal hernias, coronary artery thickening, angina pectoris, myocardial infarction, decreased joint mobility, and frequent infections. X-rays show bony abnormalities, including small, wedged-shaped vertebrae. The condition can be diagnosed *in utero* by assay of α-L-iduronidase in the fetal blood.

Hutchinson-Gilford syndrome

Other name Progeria

Hutchinson-Gilford syndrome is a very rare disease of young children; it is possibly inherited as an autosomal recessive disorder. The child has a very old appearance, which can be partly present at birth, or develops within the first 10 years of life. The face is prematurely wrinkled, with small jaws, often protruding eyes, enlarged scalp veins, and sparse growth of hair. Later features are premature graying of the hair and alopecia, growth stagnation, and arteriosclerosis. Intelligence is usually normal. Affected people usually die before the age of 20 years from the effects of arteriosclerosis.

Hyaline membrane disease

Hyaline membrane disease is characterized pathologically by lining of the distant respiratory bronchioles with hyaline membrane, composed of plasma exudation products and necrotic epithelium, pulmonary atelectasis, congestion, and edema. The birth of the affected child is usually premature. Clinical features are respiratory distress, cyanosis, a characteristic grunt during expiration, hypotension, hypothermia, pulmonary edema, and peripheral edema. There is a deficiency of surfactant. Death can occur within the first 5 days of life, but if the infant survives beyond that time, there should be a gradual improvement.

Hydrancephaly

Hydrancephaly is a condition in which the cerebral hemispheres and corpus striatum are largely replaced by a membranous sac of glial tissue containing cerebrospinal fluid. The basal ganglia, brainstem and cerebellum may be present, but show abnormalities. The child is likely to present with irritability, continuous crying when awake, feeding problems, increased muscle tone, and optic atrophy. Death within 2–3 months of birth is likely.

Hydrocele, congenital

Congenital hydrocele is present in nearly 2% of male neonates. It is usually associated with a patent ductus vaginalis. The ductus vaginalis usually closes in the first or second year of life. It can persist in 15–20% of boys. An inguinal hernia can be an associated condition.

Hydrocephalus

Hydrocephalus is an abnormal accumulation of cerebrospinal fluid with enlargement of the ventricles, atrophy of the brain and mental deterioration. As a single condition, it occurs in about 1 in 1700 live births. It is commonly associated with spina bifida. About one-third of cases are due to a congenital stenosis of the aqueduct. As an X-linked condition, it is associated with aqueduct stenosis, absence or hypoplasia of the pyramids, adducted flexed thumbs, and mental retardation.

Hydrocolpos

Hydrocolpos is an accumulation of fluid in an obstructed vagina. The obstruction may be an imperforate hymen or, less commonly, a transverse vaginal septum or vaginal atresia. It can cause urinary obstruction.

Hydrolethalus

Hydrolethalus syndrome is an autosomal recessive condition characterized by multiple abnormalities such as hydrocephalus, micrognathia, polydactyly, congenital heart disease, hypoplastic or malformed larynx, cleft palate and lip, duplicated uterus in females, and hypospadias in males. The mother's pregnancy may have been complicated by polyhydramnios or preterm delivery. Many patients are stillborn, and survivors are likely to die in the postnatal period.

Hydrometrocolpos

Hydrometrocolpos is an accumulation of fluid in the uterus and vagina due to a vaginal obstruction. The obstruction may be due to an imperforate hymen or, less commonly, to a vaginal septum or vaginal atresia. It can present as a lower abdominal mass and cause urinary tract obstruction.

Hydronephrosis

Hydronephrosis is a dilatation of the renal pelvis. It is usually associated with dilatation of the calyces of the kidney. The common causes are obstruction at the pelvic–ureteral junction or an abnormality of the vesicoureteral junction with reflux. The condition can arise in the fetus, with back pressure from retained fetal urine liable to cause irreversible renal damage. The neonate may present an abdominal mass, usually in the flank. Sepsis is a complication. Associated conditions can be an absent or defective abdominal wall, vertebral abnormalities, hypospadias and bony abnormalities.

Hydrops fetalis

Hydrops fetalis is a generalized edema of the neonate. It can vary from slight edema to massive edema with pleural and pericardial effusions and ascites. In severe cases, death occurs *in utero* or shortly after birth. Pathological causes can be anemia, low colloid pressure with hypoproteinemia, and congestive heart failure with hypervolemia. It is a feature of many congenital disorders.

3-Hydroxy-3-methylglutaryl-CoA lyase deficiency

3-Hydroxy-3-methylglutaryl-CoA lyase deficiency is an autosomal condition due to a block in the final enzyme of the leucine catabolic pathway. Prenatal diagnosis can be made. Clinical features, which develop in the neonatal period, are lethargy, hypotonia, vomiting, metabolic acidosis and coma.

Hyperammonemia of the newborn

Hyperammonemia of the newborn is a condition in which the blood ammonium concentration is raised and other laboratory findings are normal. The cause is unknown. The hyperammonemia develops within the first 24 h of life. Clinical features are hypotonia, lethargy, and coma. Without adequate treatment, death is likely in the neonatal period.

Hyperargininemia
See Urea cycle disorders

Hyperglycinemia, acute neonatal non-ketotic

Acute neonatal non-ketotic hyperglycinemia is a form of hyperglycinemia which seems to be due to a defect in the glycine cleavage enzyme. After being apparently normal at birth and for 24–36 h thereafter, the child becomes hypotonic and unresponsive and, on the third or fourth day, has generalized fits. The liver is not enlarged. The blood glycine level is increased, and the cerebrospinal fluid level of glycine can be increased 20–40 times above the normal. There is no effective treatment and the affected child can die within a few weeks or survive with severe neurological deterioration and myoclonic fits.

Hypermethioninemia

Methionine adenosyltransferase deficiency can occur, with elevated concentrations of methionine in the blood. It is an autosomal recessive condition. Most children with the condition appear normal; others can develop fatty liver, proximal muscle weakness and mental retardation.

Hyperparathyroidism

Congenital hyperparathyroidism is characterized by serum calcium levels of 15–30 mg/dl and a serum inorganic phosphate level below 3.5 mg/dl. It is characterized by anemia, enlargement of the liver and spleen, elfin facies, depressed sternum, kyphosis, renal calcinosis, and fractures. It can be associated with familial hypocalciuric hypercalcemia, and it can be a feature of multiple endocrine adenomatosis syndrome.

Hypochondroplasia

Hypochondroplasia is an autosomal dominant condition characterized by short stature, short limbs, short fingers and toes, bowing of the legs, caudal narrowing of the spine, and, sometimes, cataract, ptosis, and mental retardation. The head and face are normal or nearly normal.

Hypoglossia–hypodactylia syndrome

Hypoglossia–hypodactylia syndrome is a congenital syndrome characterized by a short or absent tongue and short or absent digits.

Hypohidrotic ectodermal dysplasia

Hypohidrotic ectodermal dysplasia is an X-linked recessive condition in which the sweat and sebaceous glands are hypoplastic or absent, with an absence of sweating and, in consequence, the development of hyperthermia. Other features can be thin, hypoplastic skin, absence of mucous glands in the oral, nasal and bronchial mucosa, absence or poor development of teeth, and absence or poor development of mammary glands.

Hypoparathyroidism

Congenital hypoparathyroidism is usually a transient condition associated with maternal diabetes mellitus, prematurity and perinatal asphyxia. Permanent congenital hypoparathyroidism is rare and is due to a failure of development of the parathyroid glands, which is due to defective embryogenesis in the third to fourth pharyngeal pouches; it presents with dysmorphic facies and severe growth failure.

Hypophosphatasia

Hypophosphatasia (with an abnormally low serum level of alkaline phosphatase) can occur congenitally. Clinical features are likely to be small stature, poor mineralization of the skeleton, bowing of long bones, short ribs, small thoracic cage, respiratory insufficiency, failure to thrive, and death in early infancy.

Hypoplastic left heart syndrome

In hypoplastic left heart syndrome, the left ventricle, mitral valve, aortic valve and ascending aorta are absent or underdeveloped. The right ventricle, as well as supplying the pulmonary circulation, supplies part of the ascending aorta, the arch of the aorta, and the descending aorta via a patent ductus arteriosus. The child usually does not live for more than a few days.

See also Heart malformations

Hypospadias

Hypospadias is a congenital deformity of the urethra, the anterior part of which is incompletely formed. In males, the opening of the urethra is on the underside of the penis or on the perineum. Inguinal hernia and cryptorchidism may be present. In females, the opening is into the vagina.

Hypospadias–dysphagia syndrome
See Opitz–Frias syndrome

I

IBIDS syndrome

IBIDS syndrome is an autosomal recessive disorder characterized by:
I – ichthyosis
B – brittle hair
I – impairment (physical and mental)
D – decreased fertility
S – short stature

See also BIDS syndrome

Ichthyosis hystrix

Ichthyosis hystrix is a form of epidermal nevi in which the lesions appear as whorls, feathery streaks, sheets or marbling of the skin. They usually involve both sides of the body, but in some patients, they stop in the midline.

Idiopathic left heart syndrome

Idiopathic left heart syndrome is characterized by hypoplasia of the left ventricle with a diminutive outflow tract, aortic valve and ascending aorta. It is often associated with a large patent ductus arteriosus and pulmonary hypertension.

See also Heart malformations

IgA deficiency

Deficiency of immunoglobulin A (IgA) is the most common primary immunodeficiency, with an incidence of about 1 in 600 people of European descent. It is much less common in Japanese and Malayans. In some people, it can be symptomless. Others are likely to have recurrent infections of the upper respiratory tract, bronchiectasis, mucocutaneous candidiasis, chronic gastrointestinal infection, allergic disorders (eczema, asthma, urticaria, allergic conjunctivitis, rhinitis, food allergies), autoimmune disorders (rheumatoid arthritis, systemic lupus erythematosus, hemolytic anemias, chronic nephritis, Sjögren's syndrome, sarcoidosis, etc.), gastrointestinal disorders (celiac disease, pancreatic insufficiency, disaccharidase deficiency, regional enteritis, ulcerative colitis), nodular lymphoid hyperplasia, pernicious anemia, cholelithiasis, chronic active hepatitis, primary biliary cirrhosis, pyoderma granulosum, hemorrhagic purpura, and Henoch-Schönlein syndrome. There is an increased liability to develop tumors. Ataxia telangiectasia is an associated condition.

Immature lung syndrome

Other name Primary atelectasis

Immature lung syndrome is incomplete expansion of the lungs due to their failure to expand at birth, or to collapse of pulmonary alveoli soon after birth. Associated conditions are immaturity, recurrent collapse of the lower lobes of the lungs, a hypoplastic pulmonary artery, and diaphragmatic hernia.

Immotile cilia syndrome

Other names Ciliary dyskinesia; Kartagener syndrome; Afzelius syndrome

Immotile cilia syndrome is an autosomal inherited disorder in which there is an absence of the dyenin arms of cilia, arms which are essential for the mobility of cilia, dyenin being a substance that can convert chemical energy into tubular contractility. Principal effects are on (1) ciliated cells of the respiratory system, with a liability to develop bronchitis and bronchiectasis, and (2) spermatozoa, whose tails are affected and movement limited, with the production of infertility in male patients. Sinus inversus (lateral transposition of the thoracic and abdominal organs) or dextrocardia can be present. The mobility of polymorphonuclear leukocytes is diminished. Other features can be chronic otitis media, sinusitis, and recurrent infections, with *Pneumococcus* and *Haemophilus* as the common infecting microorganisms.

Immunodeficiency with hyper-IgM

Immunodeficiency with hyper-immunoglobulin (Ig)M is a rare disorder characterized by low or absent IgA and IgG, and low or increased serum levels of IgM and IgD. Lymph nodes show an absence of germinal centers. There may be a concurrent T-cell deficiency. Primary and secondary forms exist.

Clinical features of the primary form include infection of the upper respiratory tract, pneumonia, otitis, oral ulcers, stomatitis, diarrhea, enlarged liver and spleen, arthritis, and an increased incidence of tumors.

The secondary form has been associated with rubella, chronic pulmonary infections, autoimmune hemolytic anemia, tumors, and anti-epileptic drugs. Clinical features include pneumonia, sepsis, recurrent infections, anemia, and enlarged liver and spleen.

See also X-linked immunodeficiency with hyper-IgM.

Incontinentia pigmenti
See Bloch–Sulzberger syndrome

Inguinal hernia

Inguinal hernia occurs in 3% of normally developed infants, in 10% of infants with low birth weight, and in 40% of infants with very low birth weight. The risk is increased by intrauterine growth retardation. The hernia can become incarcerated.

Intestinal duplications

Duplications of the intestine are rare. The usual site is the small intestine, with most attached to the ileum. They can be spherical or globular. They usually lie on the mesenteric side of the bowel, with which they share the blood supply. They are lined with intestinal mucosa. There can be an opening between the bowel and the duplication. Clinical features can be vomiting, an abdominal mass, and signs of obstruction.

Intestinal hepatodiaphragmatic interposition

Other name Chilaiditi syndrome

Chilaiditi syndrome is a condition in which part of the intestine is interposed between the liver and the right dome of the diaphragm. It can occur transiently (sliding type), but adhesions can cause it to be persistent. The hepatic flexure of the colon is the commonest part of the intestine to be interposed, but part of the small intestine and the omentum can be there. It can be asymptomatic or present with abdominal tenderness, diffuse abdominal pain, nausea, vomiting, flatulence, constipation, shortness of breath, substernal pain, and displacement of the liver.

Intestinal malrotation

Intestinal malrotation occurs in about 1 in 6000 births. It develops between the 8th and 10th week of fetal life, at a time when the intestine re-enters the abdominal cavity. If the mesenteric attachments do not develop correctly, the midgut, being attached at one end to the duodenum and at the other to the colon, is free to twist in either direction, and may twist several times. The duodenal junction can then become obstructed and, if the circulation is obstructed, the bowel becomes gangrenous. Symptoms of obstruction develop at about 1 month of life.

Intracranial angiomas

Intracranial angiomas are congenital lobulated masses consisting of large and small blood-containing spaces. They can bleed, and there is an association with epilepsy.

Intracranial arteriovenous malformations

Intracranial arteriovenous malformations are congenital abnormalities of vascular development consisting of masses of enlarged and tortuous veins and arteries in many different sizes, anastomoses and sites. They are usually supplied by one or more large arteries and drain into one or more large veins. There may be communications from the middle meningeal, superficial temporal and occipital arteries. The most common sites are in the area supplied by the middle cerebral artery and the brainstem. There is a liability to bleed, causing intracerebral or subarachnoid hemorrhage. There can be increased vascularity of the scalp, with large, pulsating arteries and hypertrophy of the carotid arteries, with a bruit being heard over them. Secondary cardiac hypertrophy can be present.

Intracranial capillary angioma

Other name Capillary telangiectasia

Intracranial capillary angioma is a congenital lesion composed of greatly dilated capillaries. The pons is a common site. Rupture can cause death. They can be associated with Osler–Pendu–Vaquez disease (hereditary hemorrhagic telangiectasia).

Isolated dextrocardia

Isolated dextrocardia is dextrocardia with the abdominal organs in the normal position. It is associated with severe cardiac malformations, such as single ventricle, ventricular inversion or pulmonary stenosis.

See also Heart malformations

Isolated levocardia

Isolated levocardia has the heart in normal position with partial or complete transposition of the abdominal organs. It is usually associated with severe cardiac malformations.

See also Heart malformations

Isovaleric acidemia

Other name Sweaty-foot syndrome

Isovaleric acidemia is an autosomal recessive condition in which there is a defect in the leucine metabolic pathway, and isovaleric acid is present in blood, cerebrospinal fluid and urine. Metabolic acidosis is apparent in the neonatal period and the infant develops lethargy, vomiting and weight loss. There is an offensive odor of rancid cheese or dried sweat given off from the skin. If inadequately treated, the child can become mentally retarded or die in an acute metabolic crisis precipitated by an infection.

Ivemark syndrome
See Asplenia syndrome

J

Jackson-Weiss syndrome

Jackson-Weiss syndrome is characterized by craniosynostosis, mid-facial hypoplasia, and abnormalities of the feet.

Jarcho-Levin syndrome

Other name Spondylothoracic dysplasia

Jarcho-Levin syndrome is an autosomal recessive condition characterized by multiple vertebral defects, short ribs, and small chest. Other features can be anal atresia, urethral atresia, bilobed bladder, ureteral obstruction, uterus didelphys, and absent external genitalia. Most affected infants die of respiratory insufficiency in the first year of life.

Jejunoileal atresia

Jejunoileal atresia is a complete obstruction of the jejunum or ileum, probably due to failure of recanalization during the 8-10th week of fetal life. There may be a history of maternal hydramnios. Clinical features are likely to be bilious vomiting, abdominal distension, failure to pass meconium, and jaundice. Associated features can be other extra-intestinal abnormalities. Unlike duodenal atresia, it is not common in Down syndrome.

Jervell-Lange-Nielsen syndrome

Other names Surdocardiac syndrome; cardioauditory syndrome

Jervell-Lange-Nielsen syndrome is an autosomal recessive disorder characterized by congenital deaf mutism and a long Q-T interval on an electrocardiogram. The etiology is unknown. The long Q-T interval is thought to be due to a congenital anomaly of myocardial metabolism, with delay of the repolarization phase, due to an enzyme deficiency. No gross abnormality of the heart is present. Paroxysmal ventricular fibrillation or tachycardia and fainting fits can occur. Sudden death in early childhood is likely.

Jeune syndrome

Other name Asphyxiating thoracic dysplasia

Jeune syndrome is an autosomal recessive condition characterized by short stature, short limbs, small thoracic cage, pulmonary hypoplasia, cystic disease of the kidney, chronic nephritis, nephronophthisis, and, sometimes, retinal degeneration, polydactyly, and pancreatic cysts. Death in infancy is likely, due to asphyxial attacks or renal failure.

Johanson–Blizzard syndrome

Johanson–Blizzard syndrome is an autosomal recessive disorder characterized by prenatal growth deficiency, microcephaly, midline posterior scalp defects, hypoplastic alae nasi, hypoplastic primary dentition, and absent secondary dentition, hypothyroidism, pancreatic deficiency, malabsorption, imperforate anus, septate or double vagina in females, and small penis and cryptorchidism in males. Patients may be intelligent or mentally retarded.

Juberg–Haward syndrome

See Oro–cranio–digital syndrome

Jugular lymphatic obstruction

In the fetus, at about the 40th day, the jugular lymphatic sac should open into the internal jugular vein. If this opening does not develop, the internal jugular sac becomes distended, the skin over it enlarges and peripheral lymphedema forms, veins become enlarged, the skin becomes overgrown, and the condition becomes lethal if no communication develops by mid-fetal life. If it does develop, the swelling subsides, skin folds appear (pterygium colli), and at birth, the hands and feet may be puffy. The condition can occur in a number of congenital disorders, including Turner syndrome. A similar condition can occur in the legs and external genitalia if there is an obstruction or delay in the development of communication between the iliac lymph sacs and the venous system. Prune belly syndrome can be an associated condition.

Juvenile xanthogranuloma

Juvenile xanthogranuloma are granulomas (benign tumors of fat-laden histiocytic cells, giant cells, and chronic inflammatory tissue) which can be present at birth, in the skin of the upper part of the body. They present as yellowish-red nodules or papules. Ocular tumors can develop.

K

Karsch–Neugebauer syndrome

Karsch–Neugebauer syndrome is a congenital condition due to the action of a single dominant gene, with marked variability of expression and incomplete penetrance. It is characterized by lobster claw malformation of the hand and foot, and nystagmus.

Kartagener syndrome
See Immotile cilia syndrome

Kast syndrome
See Maffucci syndrome

Kaufman oculocerebrofacial syndrome

Kaufman oculocerebrofacial syndrome is usually an autosomal recessive condition, but it can be sporadic and autosomal dominant. Clinical features are microcephaly, blepharophymosis, eyes with mongolian slant, micrognathia, a projecting thin upper lip, and mental retardation.

Kenny–Caffey syndrome

Kenny–Caffey syndrome is an autosomal dominant condition characterized by short stature, myopia, microphthalmia, cortical thickening of bone, thin medullary bone cavities, anemia, and transient hypocalcemia.

Keratitis, ichthyosis, deafness syndrome

Other name KID syndrome

Keratitis, ichthyosis, deafness syndrome is characterized by keratitis which can go on to blindness, ichthyosis of fine scales and follicular hyperkeratosis, and neurosensory deafness. Associated conditions are decreased or absent sweat secretion, and frequent infections.

Keutel syndrome

Keutel syndrome is an autosomal recessive condition characterized by hypoplasia of the mid-face, abnormally short distal phalanges of the fingers, calcification in the tracheobronchial tract, nose and ears, and hearing impairment.

KID Syndrome

See Keratitis, ichthyosis, deafness syndrome

Killian/Teschler–Nicola syndrome

See Pallister syndrome

Kinky hair disease

See Menkes syndrome

Klinefelter syndrome

Other name XXY syndrome

In Klinefelter syndrome, an additional X chromosome (XXY karyotype) is associated with primary testicular failure. The incidence is about 1.3 per 1000 male births. Common features are tall stature, slim build, poor sexual development, small, hard testes, gynecomastia and infertility. Other features can be cryptorchidism, hypospadias and, in later life, chronic bronchitis and diabetes mellitus. Intelligence is varied and related to the family intelligence, with the majority of patients being of average intelligence. Some have learning difficulties and delayed speech development.

Klippel–Feil syndrome

Klippel–Feil syndrome is a reduction in the number of cervical vertebrae or the fusion of multiple cervical hemivertebrae, causing shortness or stiffness of the neck and a low hair-line. Other features can be paraplegia, hemiplegia, cranial and spinal nerve palsies, and a liability of fracture of the cervical part of the spinal column.

Klippel–Trenaunay syndrome

See Klippel–Trenaunay–Weber syndrome

Klippel–Trenaunay–Weber syndrome

Other names Klippel–Trenaunay syndrome; osteohypertrophic angioectases

Klippel–Trenaunay–Weber syndrome is characterized by multiple malformations of soft tissue and bone, including arteriovenous aneurysms, cutaneous telangiectasia, vascular hamartomas, syndactyly, polydactyly, and cleft palate. Hypertrophy of bones and soft tissues occurs as a result of the increased flow of blood to the limbs. An arteriovenous shunt can lead to the development of high-output heart failure. The patient can have a wide, short neck and may be unable to extend it; this can be an anesthesiology problem.

Kniest syndrome

Kniest syndrome is probably an autosomal dominant condition. It is characterized by short stature, barrel-shaped chest, flat facies, cleft palate, short limbs, enlarged joints with stiffness, discomfort and restricted mobility, lumbar kyphoscoliosis, umbilical and inguinal hernia, and platyspondyly.

Kostmann syndrome

Other name Agranulocytosis

Kostmann syndrome is a congenital disorder characterized by severe neutropenia and maturation arrest at the myelocyte level. It runs a progressively downhill course with death usually within the first year of life, and usually from pulmonary infection with *Pseudomonas* or *Staphylococcus aureus*.

Kozlowski syndrome

Other name Spondylometaphyseal dysplasia

Kozlowski syndrome is an autosomal dominant condition with most cases representing fresh mutations. It is characterized by growth deficiency, short neck, odontoid hypoplasia, short trunk, flattened vertebrae, dorsal kyphosis, rachitic-like metaphyses, and limited joint mobility.

L

Lacrimo-auriculo-dento-digital syndrome
See Levy-Hollister syndrome

LAMB syndrome

LAMB syndrome is characterized by:
L – lentigenes (freckles)
A – atrial myxoma
M – mucous myxomas
B – blue nevi
It may be the same as NAME syndrome.

Langer-Gideon syndrome

Langer-Gideon syndrome is one of the contiguous gene syndromes. There is a combination of mental retardation and multiple physical abnormalities, including microcephaly, protruding ears, large bulbous nose, multiple exostoses of long bones, syndactyly, lax joints, and loose redundant skin. There is a deletion of chromosome 8q in 25% of affected people.

Langer mesomelic dysplasia

Langer mesomelic dysplasia is an autosomal dominant condition characterized by short stature, short forearms and lower limbs, bowed short radius, short ulna, and a rudimentary fibula.

Langer-Saldino syndrome
See Achondrogenesis type II

Laron syndrome

Laron syndrome is a primary growth hormone resistance disease. It is characterized by extremely short stature, lack of growth in lower limbs, prominent forehead, saddle nose, small hands and feet, small genitalia, small gonads, and, later in life, obesity. There is a high concentration of circulating growth hormone in the blood and very low concentration of insulin-like growth factor I.

Larsen syndrome

Larsen syndrome is an autosomal dominant disorder characterized by a flat face, hypertelorism, and a liability to multiple dislocations of joints. The soft palate can be cleft and cervical vertebrae can show abnormal segmentation.

Laryngeal atresia

Congenital laryngeal atresia is obstruction of the larynx by a web, which causes severe respiratory obstruction and cyanosis. Other serious congenital malformations may be present.

Laryngeal stridor

Congenital laryngeal stridor is a loud inspiratory stridor with chest retraction due to prolapse of the epiglottis, arytenoid cartilages and aryepiglottic folds. It improves if the infant is placed in the supine position with the neck extended.

Laryngo-tracheo-esophageal cleft

Laryngo-tracheo-esophageal cleft is a longitudinal opening between the trachea and larynx and the esophagus. Food and saliva can pass into the larynx and trachea with the production of aspiration pneumonia. Other features can be cyanosis and respiratory distress.

Lateral cervical cysts
See Branchial cysts

Laurence-Moon-Biedl syndrome

Laurence-Moon-Biedl syndrome is an autosomal recessive inherited condition characterized by obesity, gonadal hypoplasia and retinitis pigmentosa. Associated conditions can be spastic paraplegia, congenital heart defects, polydactyly, syndactyly, skull defects, diabetes mellitus and mental retardation.

Left colon syndrome

Left colon syndrome is a colonic obstruction in the newborn due to contraction of the left colon from the splenic flexure downwards. If untreated, cecal perforation can occur. Associated conditions are toxemia of pregnancy, exchange perfusion, and maternal diabetes mellitus. Immature neurons have been described in the wall of the descending colon.

Lenz syndrome

Lenz syndrome is an X-linked recessive syndrome characterized by microphthalmos, coloboma, dysmorphic ears, short stature, and mental retardation.

Lenz–Majewski hyperostosis syndrome

Lenz–Majewski hyperostosis syndrome is characterized by progressive hyperostosis, large head, prominent forehead, hypertelorism, large fontanels, syndactyly and cutis laxa. Death occurs in childhood or adolescence.

LEOPARD syndrome

LEOPARD syndrome is an autosomal dominant inherited disorder characterized by:
L – lentigenes (freckles) on the head and neck
E – electrocardiographic conduction abnormalities
O – ocular hypertelorism
P – pulmonary stenosis
A – abnormal genitalia
R – retardation of growth
D – deafness (sensorineural)
Other features can be abnormal pigmentation of the iris and retina, subaortic stenosis, hypertrophic cardiomyopathy, unilateral renal hypoplasia or agenesis, unilateral testicular or ovarian hypoplasia, and mental retardation. Lentigenes may not be present.

Leprechaunism
See Donohue syndrome

Leri–Weill syndrome

Other name Dyschondrosteosis

Leri–Weill syndrome is an autosomal dominant condition characterized by short forearms, bowing of radius, short stature, short lower
leg, and, sometimes, short hands and feet and other bony abnormalities.

Leroy I-cell syndrome

Other name Mucolipoidosis II

Leroy I-cell syndrome is an autosomal recessive condition in which
there is an increase of lysosomal enzymes in plasma, cerebrospinal
fluid and urine or an increase in serum activity of β-hexosaminidase,
iduronate sulfatase, and arylsulfatase A. It is characterized by prenatal growth deficiency, alveolar ridge hypertrophy, joint limitation,
especially of the hips, wrists and fingers, thick tight skin, slight
enlargement of the liver, and separation of the recti abdominalis
muscles.

Lethal multiple pterygium syndrome

Lethal multiple pterygium syndrome is a fatal autosomal recessive
condition in which the child is stillborn or dies shortly after birth.
It is characterized by multiple pterygia (abnormal folds of skin and
fascia) in the neck and elsewhere, flexion contractures of shoulders,
elbows, hands, hips, knees, ankles and feet, hypertelorism, flat nose,
cryptorchidism, and cardiac and pulmonary hypoplasia.

Leukocyte adhesion deficiency

Leukocyte adhesion deficiency is a severe congenital immunodeficiency, due to a deficiency in leukocyte β_2 integrins. Clinical features
are the persistence of a 'fleshy', often infected, umbilical stump,
delayed wound healing, and recurrent and often fatal infections.

Levy–Hollister syndrome

Other name Lacrimo–auriculo–dento–digital syndrome

Levy–Hollister syndrome is an autosomal dominant condition
characterized by nasolacrimal duct obstruction, external ear deformities, deafness, absence of some of the teeth, enamel hypoplasia of
primary and secondary dentitions, and abnormalities of radius, ulna,
thumb and fingers.

Lewis syndrome

Other name Upper limb cardiovascular syndrome

Lewis syndrome is an autosomal dominant condition in which multiple skeletal abnormalities of the upper limb are associated with congenital heart disease and disturbances of atrial and ventricular cardiac conduction.

Limb-body wall syndrome

Limb-body wall syndrome can be a feature of early amnion rupture syndrome when the extraembryonic celom persists after the normal 60 days. The amnion becomes attached abnormally to the head, chest and abdomen. Features can be anencephaly, oblique facial clefts, encephaloceles, ventral wall defect, thoracoschisis, evisceration, and constriction rings of the digits.

See also Early amnion rupture syndrome

Lindau-Hippel syndrome
See Hippel-Lindau syndrome

Linear nevus sebaceus syndrome
See Fuerstein-Mimms syndrome

Linear sebaceous nevus

Other name Nevus sebaceus of Jadassohn

Linear sebaceus nevus is a congenital lesion usually of the mid-facial region, but sometimes on the trunk and limbs, associated with convulsions and mental retardation.

Lipomeningomyelocele
See under Spina bifida cystica

Lip pit-cleft lip syndrome
See Van Der Woude syndrome

Lip pit syndrome
See Demarquay syndrome

Lissencephaly

Lissencephaly is a hypoplasia of the brain characterized by complete or partial absence of gyri. The cortex may be completely smooth or there may be some sulci and poorly developed gyri. It can be due to primary agenesis or to secondary destruction of the cortex at any early stage of development. Other features can be hypoplasia or absence of the corpus callosum, small brainstem, microcephaly, a high forehead with vertical ridges and furrows, abnormal electroencephalogram (EEG), epilepsy, and severe mental retardation. Other features can be cardiac defects, cryptorchidism, piloidal sinus, and failure to thrive. Death occurs in childhood, often before the age of 3 months. Type I lissencephaly is the most severe form, with a thick cortex and maximal developmental arrest; it can be sporadic or be a feature of Miller–Dieker syndrome, which is associated with a deletion on chromosome 17. Type II lissencephaly has a thin disorganized cortex and is a feature of Walker–Warburg syndrome.

'Lobster claw' defect
See Ectrodactyly

Loose anagen syndrome

Loose anagen syndrome is a congenital disorder of hair. Hair is short and sparse, grows slowly, seldom requires cutting, and pulls out easily. There is in consequence a patchy, diffuse alopecia. Light microscopy of the hair roots shows distorted anagen bulbs, rolled-back cuticle scales, and absent outer root sheaths. The condition improves with age. There are no other congenital abnormalities.

Lop ear
See External ear disorders

Lowe syndrome

Other name Oculocerebrorenal syndrome

Lowe syndrome is an X-linked recessive disorder characterized by mental retardation, small eyes, congenital cataracts, congenital glaucoma, strabismus, buphthalmos, hypotonia, absent tendon reflexes, fits, osteoporosis, and a renal tubular defect which causes proteinuria, amine aciduria and acidosis.

M

Macrocephaly

Macrocephaly is an abnormally large brain. It can be an isolated condition or it can be part of a general growth disorder (such as Sotos syndrome) or part of a neurological disorder.

Macroglossia

Macroglossia is enlargement of the tongue, with its protrusion from the mouth. It can be due to idiopathic hypertrophy of the muscle, lymphangioma, or the presence of thyroid tissue as a cystic or solid tumor in the tongue, due to a failure of migration of the thyroid gland; there may be no other thyroid tissue in the neck. Macroglossia is commonly a feature of Down syndrome and Beckwith syndrome.

Majewski syndrome

Other name Short rib–polydactyly syndrome II

Majewski syndrome is an autosomal recessive condition characterized by short limbs and ribs, a narrow chest, polydactyly, cleft lip or palate, heart defects, renal cysts and genital abnormalities.

Major histocompatibility complex class II-deficient combined immunodeficiency

Major histocompatibility complex class II-deficient combined immunodeficiency is a condition in which patients without these molecules have abnormal cellular and humoral responses to specific antigen and are liable to have severe and repeated infections. These infections are likely to be intestinal infections, severe viral infections, and respiratory tract infections and to cause death in infancy and early childhood.

Malignant melanoma

Malignant melanoma can arise transplacentally from the mother and be present at birth in any part of the body. The placenta may have a brown-black color with malignant cells in the intervillous spaces and cord blood.

Mandibulo-facial dyscephaly

See Hallermann–Streiff syndrome

Maple syrup urine disease

Maple syrup urine disease is an autosomal recessive condition in which there is an error of metabolism involving leucine, isoleucine and valine. In the severe form of the disease, on the second or third day of life, the infant becomes lethargic and then starts to vomit, feeds poorly, loses weight, and, later, develops hypertonia or hypotonia and seizures, and, without adequate treatment, dies. In less severe forms, in which there is some enzyme activity, the infant appears normal during the neonatal period and demonstrates features of the disease in infancy or childhood.

Marfan syndrome

Marfan syndrome is an autosomal dominant disorder due to mutations of the fibrillin gene on chromosome 15. It is a disorder of collagen. Clinical features are asthenic build, tall stature, long arms and legs, arachnodactyly, highly arched palate, kyphoscoliosis, and easily dislocated joints. Other features can be cataracts, detachment of the retina, and dislocation of the lens before the age of 12 years (the suspensory ligaments are at the wrong tension, owing to the eyes being too long), aortic regurgitation, mitral regurgitation, coronary thromboses, pneumothorax, and often a fatal dissecting aneurysm of the aorta. Schizophrenia can be an associated condition.

Marchesani syndrome

Marchesani syndrome is an autosomal recessive disorder with multiple skeletal and ocular deformities. An affected patient is short and stocky with well developed muscles. The hands and feet are spade-shaped. X-rays show delayed carpal and tarsal ossification. Ocular abnormalities include ectopia lentis (displacement of the lens of the eye), spherophakia (spherical lens), iridodonesis (tremulousness of the iris due to lack of support by the lens), and glaucoma.

Marden–Walker syndrome

Marden–Walker syndrome is characterized by a mask-like face, micrognathia, blepharophimosis, cleft or highly arched palate, low set ears, joint contractures, kyphoscoliosis, and psychomotor retardation. Associated conditions can be heart defects, microcystic kidneys, pyloric stenosis, Zollinger–Ellison syndrome, and Dandy–Walker malformation with vertebral abnormalities.

Marinesco–Garland syndrome

See Marinesco–Sjögren syndrome

Marinesco–Sjögren syndrome

Other names Marinesco–Garland syndrome; cataract–oligophrenia syndrome

Marinesco–Sjögren syndrome is an autosomal recessive disorder characterized by cerebellar ataxia, dysarthria, short stature, abnormal teeth, cataracts, thin brittle hair, thin fragile nails, and mental retardation.

Maroteaux–Lamy syndrome

Other name Mucopolysaccharidosis VI

Maroteaux–Lamy syndrome is an autosomal recessive disorder of mucopolysaccharide metabolism due to a deficiency of the enzyme aryl sulfatase B. Clinical features are short stature, lumbar kyphosis, genu valgum, hydrocephalus, cardiac valvular disease, and, often, enlargement of the liver and spleen. Intelligence is normal or nearly normal. The patient usually survives to the 20s.

Marshall syndrome

Marshall syndrome is an autosomal dominant condition characterized by sensorineural deafness, cataracts and saddle nose.

Marshall–Smith syndrome

Marshall–Smith syndrome is characterized by accelerated skeletal maturation beginning *in utero*, long cranium, prominent forehead, prominent eyes, small mandible, broad proximal and middle phalanges, small distal phalanges, umbilical hernia, and excessive growth of hair. Other features can be macrogyria, cerebral atrophy, absent corpus callosum, and immunological deficiency. Many fail to thrive and death is common before the age of 2 years.

MASA syndrome

MASA syndrome is an X-linked condition characterized by:
M – mental retardation
A – aphasia
S – shuffling gait
A – adducted thumbs

Mastocytosis

Mastocytosis is an infiltration of mast cells in the dermis. It presents as a single lesion, a generalized maculopapular eruption, or a thickening of the skin. The single lesion is pink, yellow or brown, raised, and rubbery to the touch. Liberation of histamine from the mast cells can cause itching, flushing, irritability and tachycardia. Internal organs may be invaded by mast cells.

Maternal hyperthermia-induced syndrome

Maternal hyperthermia-induced syndrome is due to the exposure of a pregnant woman to a severe degree of hyperthermia in the first 3 months of pregnancy. Clinical features in the affected infant are likely to be microcephaly, micrognathia, mid-facial hypoplasia, cleft lip and/or palate, external ear anomalies, hypotonicity or hypertonicity, contractures, convulsions, and mental retardation.

Maternal phenylketonuria fetal syndrome

Maternal phenylketonuria can be a cause of abnormalities in the woman's children. These abnormalities can be pre- and post-natal growth deficiency, microcephaly, characteristic round facies, strabismus, congenital cardiac abnormalities, coarctation of the aorta, severe mental retardation, cerebral cortical dysfunction, convulsions, and hypertonicity. Less common features are cleft lip and palate, cervical and sacral spinal abnormalities, microphthalmia, and esophageal atresia.

Maxillary antrum abnormalities

The maxillary antrum can show bony ridges, either horizontal or vertical. A vertical ridge is usually incomplete. A horizontal ridge can divide the antrum into two cavities, the upper cavity communicating with the superior meatus, and the lower cavity with the middle meatus.

Maxillonasal dysplasia
See Binder syndrome

Mayer–Rokitansky–Küster syndrome

Other name Rokitansky–Küster–Hauser syndrome

Mayer–Rokitansky–Küster syndrome is characterized by vaginal aplasia, rudimentary cornua uteri, and morphologically normal ovaries and Fallopian tubes situated on the side wall of the pelvis. The woman is amenorrheic and infertile.

McCune–Albright syndrome
See Albright syndrome

Maffucci syndrome

Other name Kast syndrome

Maffucci syndrome is an association of cavernous hemangiomas, enchondromas, anemia, labile blood pressure, fragile bones, and sensitivity to vasodilator drugs. The hemangiomas are usually in the limbs, but they can occur in the retroperitoneal space and in the synovial membranes of joints. Complications are pathological fractures, chondrosarcoma and angiosarcoma.

Meckel diverticulum

Meckel diverticulum is present in 1.5–2% of live births. The male:female ratio is 3.5:1. The diverticulum is a persistent part of the connection between the bowel and the yolk sac, is tent-shaped or tubular, and can be 2–90 cm long. It arises from the ileum at any point within 100 cm of the cecum. The end may be free or it may be connected to the umbilicus by a fibrous cord. Rarely, it remains patent at the umbilicus with the formation of an omphalomesenteric fistula. It is normally composed of small-bowel tissue, but it can be a site of ectopic gastric or pancreatic tissue. It is usually symptomless, but the gastric mucosa in it can ulcerate, bleed and perforate just like a gastric ulcer, and the fibrous cord can cause intestinal obstruction. Inflammation of the diverticulum can cause peritonitis.

Meckel–Gruber syndrome
See Meckel syndrome

Meckel syndrome

Other name Meckel–Gruber syndrome

Meckel syndrome is an autosomal recessive condition characterized by encephalocele, hypoplasia of the olfactory lobes, microphthalmos, coloboma, cataract, cleft lip or palate, polydactyly and polycystic kidney.

Median cleft-face syndrome

Other name Frontonasal dysplasia

Median cleft-face syndrome is characterized by a split in the nose – varying in severity from completely separated nostrils to a notch in the tip of the nose – a midline defect in the frontal bone (cranium bifidum occultum), a widow's peak, and hypertelorism.

Megacalcycosis

Congenital megacalcycosis is a condition in which the calyces of the kidneys are dilated without any obstruction being present. It is more common in males than in females. It is usually asymptomatic. It may be associated with megaureter.

Megacystis megaureter
See Ureteric abnormalities

Megalencephaly

Megalencephaly is an abnormally large brain and an enlargement of the cranium, without increased intracranial pressure and widening of the sutures, and with a soft, sometimes enlarged, anterior fontanel. It can be a feature of some syndromes (Russell–Silver syndrome, Sotos syndrome, Hallermann–Streiff syndrome, Beckwith–Wiedemann syndrome) or it can occur on its own or with other anomalies. There may be no neurological symptoms, but mental retardation, fits and hypotonia can be complications.

Megaureter
See Ureteric abnormalities

MELAS syndrome

MELAS syndrome is a disorder of mitochondrial inheritance characterized by:
ME – mitochondrial encephalopathy
LA – lactic acidosis
S   – stroke-like episodes

Melnick–Fraser syndrome
See Branchio-otorenal syndrome

Melnick–Needles syndrome

Melnick–Needles syndrome is an autosomal dominant disorder which is lethal to males. Girls with the condition are characterized by prominent eyes, small mandible, short upper arms and distal phalanges, bowing of radius and tibia, short clavicles, and narrow shoulders.

Meningocele
See under Spina bifida cystica

Meningomyelocele
See under Spina bifida cystica

Menkes syndrome

Other name Kinky hair disease

Menkes syndrome is an X-linked recessive disorder associated with copper enzyme deficiency. Clinical features are sparse kinky hair, degeneration of the cerebral cortex, seborrheic dermatitis, hypopigmentation, and neurological retardation. Death from central nervous system complications can occur before 2 years of age.

Mesoblastic lymphoma

Congenital mesoblastic lymphoma is the commonest renal tumor of the newborn. Maternal polyhydramnios is an associated factor. The condition presents as a palpable mass with hematuria, hypertension, hypercalcemia, and, later, congestive heart failure.

Mesocardia

Mesocardia is a central location of the heart. The cardiac anatomy is normal and, usually, there are no congenital malformations.

Mesodermal dysgenesis

See Anterior cleavage syndrome

Metaphyseal chondrodysplasia, Jansen type

The Jansen type of metaphyseal chondrodysplasia is an autosomal dominant condition characterized by very short stature, poorly developed lower jaw, deficiency of metaphyseal ossification, small chest, flexion deformity of the knees and hips, hyperostosis of the skull, and deafness.

Metaphyseal chondrodysplasia, McKusick type

Other name Cartilage–hair hypoplasia syndrome

Metaphyseal chondrodysplasia is an autosomal recessive condition in which there is a deficiency of adenosine deaminase. Clinical features are short-limb dwarfism, dysplasia of cartilage and bone, sparse hair, redundant skin, neutropenia, defective T-cell related immunity, defective antibody production, and severe combined immunodeficiency. Death is likely before 20 years of age.

Metaphyseal chondrodysplasia, Schmid type

The Schmid type of metaphyseal chondrodysplasia is an autosomal dominant condition with variable expression and is characterized by short stature, bowing of tibiae, coxa vara, genu varum, limitation of full extension of the fingers, and hypoplasia of cartilage.

Metatropic dwarfism syndrome

Other name Metatropic dysplasia

Metatropic dwarfism syndrome is characterized by very short stature, early platyspondyly with scoliosis and kyphosis, short ribs, short limbs, enlarged joints with limited mobility at knee and hip, and hypoplasia of the pelvis.

Metatropic dysplasia

See Metatropic dwarfism syndrome

Methylmalonic acidemia

Methylmalonic acidemia is an autosomal recessive condition in which there is a defect in the enzyme methylmalonyl-CoA mutase and an accumulation of methylmalonic acid in the blood, cerebrospinal fluid and urine. Neonatal presentation is severe, with lethargy, poor feeding, hepatomegaly, severe metabolic acidosis, an increase in blood ammonia, and, without adequate treatment, death. A delayed form can appear in the 2nd or 3rd month of life.

Microcephaly

Microcephaly is a head circumference, as measured around the glabella and the occipital protuberance, that is more than two standard deviations below the mean for age, sex, race, and gestation. The brain may weigh as little as 500 g and show microgyria, micropolygyria, neuronal heterotopia (the presence of neuronal tissue in abnormal places), and agenesis of the corpus callosum. Microcephaly can be primary (due to anomalous development during the first 7 months of intrauterine life) or secondary (due to insults received during the last 3 months of intrauterine life or during the perinatal period). Primary microcephaly can be transmitted as an autosomal recessive condition and is associated with many genetic diseases. It can occur as a mildly dominant condition in some families. Isolated severe microcephaly with a normal face can be inherited as an autosomal recessive condition, with a recurrence risk of 10–20%. Causes of secondary microcephaly are congenital rubella, cytomegalovirus, toxoplasmosis, phenylketonuria, maternal irradiation, and some drugs. Clinical features can be spastic paralysis of the limbs, fits, hyperkinetic behavior, and mental retardation.

Micropenis

Micropenis is a normally formed penis with a length 2.5 standard deviations below the norm for the age. The penis of a newborn child when stretched should measure at least 2 cm from pubis to tip. The cause of micropenis is unknown; there may be a hypothalamic defect.

Microphthalmia

In microphthalmia the eyes are congenitally small. The incidence and possible causes are similar to those of anophthalmia.

Microtia

See under External ear disorders

Middle aortic syndrome

Middle aortic syndrome is characterized by severe narrowing of the abdominal aorta and of its visceral and renal branches. Clinical features include severe hypertension, headache, nose bleeds, chest pain, and cardiac failure. There is a high mortality rate.

Middle-ear abnormalities

Middle-ear abnormalities can be variations in size, displacement of walls, deformation of the fenestrae, and malformation of the ossicles. Congenital diminution of hearing is a result.

See also Stapes footplate fixation

Mietens syndrome

Mietens syndrome is characterized by corneal opacity, growth failure, flexion contracture of the elbows, and mental retardation.

Miller syndrome

See Postaxial acrofacial dysostosis syndrome

Miller–Dieker syndrome

Miller–Dieker syndrome is a form of lissencephaly in which there is a deletion on chromosome 17. It is characterized by lissencephaly, microcephaly, enlarged cerebral ventricles, thin upper lip, long philtrum, and a failure of development of the frontal and temporal lobes of the brain with depression in the temporal regions of the skull.

Mitral stenosis

In congenital mitral stenosis there is obstruction to the left atrial outflow, enlargement of the left atrium, hypertrophy of the heart, and, eventually, right ventricular failure. A late diastolic murmur is audible at the apex of the heart.

See also Heart malformations

Moebius syndrome

Moebius syndrome is a congenital syndrome characterized by complete or partial paralysis of the sixth and seventh cranial nerves due to hypoplasia or absence of their nuclei. There can be bilateral failure of ocular abduction or bilateral gaze palsy. Other features can be malformation of orofacial structures and limbs. In some cases there is autosomal dominant inheritance. In about half the cases there may have been previous uterine surgery or a severe event in pregnancy such as failed abortion, hyperthermia, electric shock, alcohol abuse, or prolonged rupture of the membranes, and the syndrome may be due to interruption of fetal blood supply.

Moerman syndrome

Moerman syndrome is a lethal condition characterized by dwarfism, macrocrania, hydrocephalus, agenesis of the corpus callosum, congenital heart defects, renal defects, and spondylocostal abnormalities.

Mohr syndrome

Other name Orofaciodigital syndrome II

Mohr syndrome is an autosomal recessive disorder characterized by conductive deafness, mid-line cleft of the tongue, low nasal bridge, hypoplasia of the maxilla, zygomatic arch and mandibular body, polydactyly, and partial reduplication of the big toe, first metatarsal bone, cuboid and cuneiform bones. Other features can be cleft palate, missing central incisors, and mental retardation.

Morquio syndrome

Other name Mucopolysaccharidosis IV

Morquio syndrome is an autosomal recessive disorder of mucopolysaccharides. In the A form, there is a deficiency of the enzyme galactosamine-6-sulfate sulfatase; in the B form, there is a deficiency of the enzyme β-galactosidase. Clinical features are short stature, coarse features, prominent sternum, kyphosis, genu valgum, waddling gait, and corneal opacities. Aortic incompetence can develop in later life. Intelligence may be below average. In the B form, the bone changes are slight; the odontoid process of the second cervical vertebra may be aplastic. The deformities are likely to become progressively worse. Most patients survive to early adulthood. Death may be due to cervical dislocation.

Mounier–Kuhn syndrome
See Tracheobronchomegaly

Moynahan syndrome

Moynahan syndrome is a congenital disorder characterized by short stature, mitral stenosis, and multiple symmetrical lentigenes (freckles).

Mucolipoidosis II
See Leroy I-cell syndrome

Mucolipoidosis III
See Pseudo-Hurler polydystrophy syndrome

Mucopolysaccharidoses

Mucopolysaccharidoses are a group of inherited metabolic disorders due to a deficiency of specific liposomal enzymes.

Mucopolysaccharidosis Ih
See Hurler syndrome

Mucopolysaccharidosis Is
See Scheie syndrome

Mucopolysaccharidosis II
See Hunter syndrome

Mucopolysaccharidosis III
See Sanfilippo syndrome

Mucopolysaccharidosis IV
See Morquio syndrome

Mucopolysaccharidosis V
See Scheie syndrome

Mucopolysaccharidosis VI
See Maroteaux–Lamy syndrome

Mucopolysaccharidosis VII
See Sly syndrome

Mulibrey-nanism syndrome
See Perheentupa syndrome

Multicystic kidney

Multicystic kidney can be detected antenatally by ultrasound. It is usually unilateral, but it can be bilateral. Unilateral kidney cysts present as a mass in the flank, and they can be associated with abdominal distension and hypertension. The renal pelvis and ureter can be absent or occluded. The contralateral kidney may be normal or show significant disease. Bilateral multicystic disease presents with anuria, pulmonary hypoplasia, Potter facies, and early death.

Multiple exostoses syndrome

Multiple exostoses syndrome is an autosomal dominant condition in which exostoses appear, usually at the ends of long bones. They are commonly present at birth and develop further in childhood. Other features can be shortness of affected bones, of stature, and of metacarpals.

Multiple synostosis syndrome

Other name Symphalangism syndrome

Multiple synostosis syndrome is an autosomal dominant condition with variance in expression. It is characterized by fusion of elbow joints, carpal and tarsal bones, and of mid-phalangeal joints. Distant phalanges are likely to be hypoplastic or aplastic. Deafness is due to fusion of middle-ear ossicles. Other features can be vertebral abnormalities and limited movement of shoulders and hips.

Multisynostotic osteodysgenesis
See Antley-Bixler syndrome

MURCS syndrome

MURCS syndrome is characterized by:
MU – Müllerian duct aplasia
R   – renal aplasia
CS – cervicothoracic somite dysplasia
Clinical features can be defects of the cervical and thoracic vertebrae, absence of the vagina, absence or hypoplasia of the uterus, primary amenorrhea, small stature, rib abnormalities, cleft lip and palate, micrognathia, and gastrointestinal abnormalities.

Myasthenia gravis

Myasthenia gravis can occur in the neonate as (a) neonatal myasthenia gravis in 10–15% of children born to myasthenic mothers and (b) congenital myasthenia gravis, myasthenia gravis in neonates born to mothers without myasthenia gravis. The child may appear normal at birth, but within hours of birth develops weakness, hypotonia, sucking difficulties, sometimes respiratory difficulties, a flat facial expression, and a weak cry. The symptoms are mild in 20%. They can persist from a few hours to several weeks.

Myodystrophia fetalis deformans

See Arthrogryposis multiplex congenita

Myotonia dystrophia

Myotonia dystrophia is an autosomal dominant condition, with a mother being the affected parent in 90% of cases. The molecular defect is an unstable DNA triplet (CTG) sequence on the long arm of chromosome 19, which is expanded. Clinical features are hypotonia, facial weakness, talipes, neonatal respiratory distress, feeding problems due to pharyngeal incoordination and palatal weakness, delayed motor development, and mental retardation. Death in the neonatal period can be due to inability to establish satisfactory respiration. There is a 25% chance of death before 18 months.

Myotonic chondrodystrophy

See Schwartz–Jampel syndrome

N

Nager syndrome

Nager syndrome is characterized by malar hypoplasia, hypoplasia of the jaws, partial or total absence of the lower eyelashes, abnormalities of the ears, cleft palate, aplasia or hypoplasia of the thumbs, short forearms, radioulnar synostosis, and limitation of extension at the elbow. Other features can be tetralogy of Fallot, hypoplastic first rib, dislocation of the hip, and club foot.

Nall-patella syndrome

Other names Turner–Kieser syndrome; Hereditary onycho-osteo-dysplasia

Nail–patella syndrome is an autosomal dominant condition in which the patellae are small or absent and nails show changes varying from ridging to absence; the thumb nails are the ones usually affected. Other anomalies can be exostoses of the ileum, malformed radial heads, and pigmentary changes in the iris. Of all sufferers from this syndrome, 40% develop renal disease, and 25% of these progress to renal failure.

NAME syndrome

NAME syndrome is characterized by:
N – nevi
A – atrial myxoma
M – myxoid neurofibromas
E – ephelides (freckles)
It may be the same as LAMB syndrome.

Nance–Horan syndrome

Nance–Horan syndrome is an X-linked congenital condition characterized by cataracts, peg-shaped and rudimentary teeth, and in about 20% of cases by broad or short fingers, developmental delay, and mental retardation.

Nasal abnormalities

Absence
Complete or partial absence of the nose is very rare.

Anterior naris atresia
One anterior naris can be occluded by a web of skin at the mucocutaneous junction. The web can be partial or complete, thin or thick and fleshy. Partial atresia can occur as a narrowing of the nasal entrance. Cleft lip can be an associated condition.

Triple nares
Triple nares are very rare. There can be two separate openings on one side, one of which can end blindly, with normal nares on the other side.

Median fissure
A median fissure is a common shallow fissure at the tip of the nose. It rarely extends into the columella (the external termination of the nasal septum).

Bifid nose
Bifid nose is a deep median fissure of varying degree of cleft, varying from simple fissure of the tip to complete separation of the anterior nares by a broad central sulcus. Cleft lip and hypertelorism can be associated conditions.

Double nose
Two noses, each with two nostrils, are present. Some of the nostrils end blindly. Hypertelorism and a dermoid cyst opening centrally above the noses can be associated conditions.

Nasolacrimal duct obstruction

Congenital obstruction of the nasolacrimal duct occurs in 1–6% of neonates and is most common in firstborn children. It is usually unilateral. It presents as a tender swelling of the skin overlying the lacrimal sac and adjacent part of the eyelid. Dacrocystitis can occur. The obstruction usually resolves spontaneously within the first 12 months of life.

Neonatal teeth

Neonatal teeth are teeth that are present at birth or erupt within the first 4 weeks of life. They can be part of the normal primary dentition or they may be supernumerary. The most common are mandibular central incisors. Most of them are firmly fixed. They can be associated with Ellis–van Creveld syndrome, Hallerman-Streiff syndrome, and pachyonychia congenita.

Neonatal withdrawal syndrome

Neonatal withdrawal syndrome is due to prolonged or repeated exposure of a child *in utero* to heroin, methadone, codeine, cocaine, meperidine, or amphetamine. It is characterized by neonatal restlessness, tremors, jitteriness, irritability, fits, hypertonicity, yawning, sweating, fever, vomiting, diarrhea, dehydration, depressed or rapid expiration, and respiratory distress.

Nephrogenic diabetes insipidus

Congenital nephrogenic diabetes insipidus is an X-linked disorder in which the kidneys are unable to concentrate urine in response to arginine vasopressin. Clinical features are passing large amounts of urine, thirst, irritability, vomiting, constipation, dehydration, fever, failure to thrive, and, later in life, mental retardation.

Netherton syndrome

Netherton syndrome is characterized by ichthyosis, defects of the hair shafts, and atopy.

Neu-Laxova syndrome

Neu–Laxova syndrome is an autosomal recessive condition. The child has microcephaly and multiple congenital deformities including atrophy of the cerebrum, cerebellum and pons, absence of the corpus callosum, hypertelorism, protruding eyes, a round, gaping mouth, syndactyly of fingers and toes, flexion contractures, scaling skin and edema. The child is stillborn or dies in the neonatal period.

Neurocutaneous melanosis

Neurocutaneous melanosis is characterized by multiple extensive nevi of the skin, usually in the abdomen, lower trunk, and upper thighs (the 'bathing trunks' area) and present at birth, melanosis of the pia-arachnoid membrane, with later convulsions, degeneration of central nervous system function, and hydrocephalus. Malignant melanoma can develop in early childhood.

Neurodermal sinus

Neurodermal sinus is a congenital sinus between the skin and the central nervous system. It is lined with squamous epithelium. The most common sites are the occipital and lumbosacral regions. Cerebrospinal fluid may drain from the sinus. Infection can enter via the sinus, and recurrent meningitis can be a complication.

Neurofibromatosis
See Recklinghausen syndrome

Nevus

Nevus is a congenital vascular malformation of the skin and mucous membranes. Many forms have been described.

Blue nevi have a deep blue color and appear in the scalp, face, arms, and buttocks.

Epidermal nevi arise in the epidermis and appear in various forms. They can be unilateral or bilateral, slightly or deeply pigmented, and well or poorly demarcated.

Giant nevi are large nevi, varying in size from several square centimeters to involving the whole body. A 'bathing trunk nevus' involves the chest, back, abdomen and upper part of the thighs.

Nevus of Ito involves the deltotrapezoid area.

Nevus of Oto is blue-gray and involves the orbital and zygomatic areas and sometimes the sclera and fundus.

Nevus flammeus (telangiectatic nevus) is common, and occurs equally in the sexes and anywhere on the skin or mucous membranes. It presents as a flat, sharply defined, bright-red or dark-red lesion. A salmon patch is a pale nevus on the forehead or between the eyes; it can have ocular complications if it occurs in the area of skin supplied by the ophthalmic branch of the trigeminal nerve.

See also Blue rubber bleb nevus syndrome; Fuerstein–Mimms syndrome; Ichthyosis hystrix; Klippel–Trenaunay–Weber syndrome; Sturge–Weber syndrome; Linear sebaceous nevus; Hoffman–Zurhette syndrome

Nevus lipomatides superficialis
See Hoffman–Zurhelle syndrome

Nevus sebaceus of Jadassohn
See Linear sebaceous nevus

Nievergelt syndrome

Nievergelt syndrome is an autosomal dominant condition and is characterized by severe shortening and deformity of the legs above the knee, sometimes shortening of the forearms, and sometimes radioulnar synostosis.

Noonan-like short stature syndrome

See Cardio–facio–cutaneous syndrome

Noonan syndrome

A patient with Noonan syndrome resembles a patient with Turner syndrome, but there is no chromosomal defect, and Noonan syndrome occurs in both sexes. In some families, there is an autosomal dominant inheritance. Clinical features are short stature, low-set ears, intelligence below average, and many minor skeletal deformities, of which the commonest are pectus excavatus amd cubitus valgus. Cerebral arteriovenous malformations may be present. Cardiac abnormalities occur in 50% of patients; these include pulmonary valve stenosis, thick and dysplastic pulmonary valves, right heart abnormalities, and left ventricular cardiomyopathy. Associated conditions can be neurofibromatosis and cherubism (familial fibrous dysplasia of the jaws).

O

Ocular–auricular–vertebral dysplasia
See Goldenhar syndrome

Oculocerebrorenal syndrome
See Lowe syndrome

Oculocutaneous albinism

Oculocutaneous albinism is a group of congenital abnormalities in which there is a defect of melanin synthesis, with hypomelanosis of the eyes, skin and hair. Associated conditions are photophobia, nystagmus, impaired visual acuity, and deafness.

Oculodentodigital syndrome

Oculodentodigital syndrome is an autosomal dominant condition with variable expression and is characterized by microphthalmos, glaucoma, hypoplastic tooth enamel, and abnormal digits. Associated features can be sensorineural deafness, cleft lip and palate, and congenital dislocation of the hip.

OEIS syndrome

OEIS syndrome is characterized by:
O – omphalocele (protrusion of intestine through umbilical defect)
E – exstrophy of the bladder
I – imperforate anus
S – spinal defect
Other abnormalities can be a failure of the pubic rami to unite, cryptorchidism and absent penis in males, and bifid uterus and vaginal atresia in females.

Oligomeganephronia
See Renal hypoplasia

Ollier syndrome

Other names Chondrodysplasia; Osteochondromatosis; Enchondromatosis

Ollier syndrome is characterized by multiple islets of unossified cartilage in the shafts of long bones. They are usually bilateral, but not symmetrical. Shortness of a limb can occur, and sometimes a tumor can be felt in a bone. Fractures are common.

Omenn syndrome

Omenn syndrome is the presence of symptoms similar to those of graft-versus-host disease in a patient with severe combined immunodeficiency. It is characterized by the presence of large numbers of T cells which are derived from a small number of T-cell clones. These T cells are present in blood, liver and spleen; the lymph nodes and thymus contain no lymphocytes. It is inherited as an autosomal recessive condition. Clinical features are erythroderma, enlargement of the liver, spleen and lymph nodes, frequent infections, and failure to thrive. Without a bone marrow transplantation, it is usually fatal in the first year of life. There can be an association with cartilage–hair hypoplasia syndrome.

Omphalocele

Omphalocele is a protrusion through a congenital defect in the formation of the umbilical and epigastric portions of the anterior abdominal wall. By definition, the defect is greater than 4 cm in diameter. An epigastric omphalocele is associated with Cantrell pentalogy (cleft sternum, lower thoracic wall malformation, defect of the diaphragm, cardiac anomaly, and pericardial defect). The mass is covered by a membrane and not by skin and subcutaneous tissue, which differentiates it from an umbilical hernia. Associated conditions can be imperforate anus and bladder exstrophy.

Opitz–Frias syndrome

Other names G syndrome; Hypospadias–dysphagia syndrome

Opitz–Frias syndrome is an autosomal dominant disorder characterized by craniofacial abnormalities, genital abnormalities, achalasia of the cardia, laryngeal hypoplasia, and functional swallowing and laryngeal difficulties. Pulmonary aspiration can occur frequently and may be fatal. Males are more severely affected than females. The condition can present difficulties for an anesthesiologist.

Ornithine transcarbamylase deficiency

See under Urea cycle disorders

Oro–cranio–digital syndrome

Other name Juberg–Hayward syndrome

Oro–cranio–digital syndrome is of uncertain inheritance; it may be recessive. It is characterized by hypertelorism, bowed upward-slanting eyelids, rib and vertebral anomalies, luxation of the radial head, short forearms, restriction of elbow movements, displacement or hypoplasia of the thumbs, horseshoe kidney, and mental retardation.

Orofaciodigital syndrome I

Orofaciodigital syndrome I is an X-linked dominant condition affecting females only. It is characterized by oral abnormalities, webbing between the alveolar ridge and mucous membrane, partial clefts in tongue and lips, cleft of soft palate, anomalous teeth (absent lateral incisors), facial abnormalities (hypoplasia of the alar cartilages, lateral placement of the inner canthi), digital abnormalities (syndactyly, short fingers, sometimes polydactyly). Other features can be agenesis of the corpus callosum, cerebral malformations, hydrocephalus, fits, and polycystic kidneys. The clinical features are similar to those of Mohr syndrome, but that syndrome is autosomal recessive, and affects both sexes.

Orofaciodigital syndrome II

See Mohr syndrome

Oromandibular-line hypogenesis syndrome

Oromandibular-line hypogenesis syndrome is a congenital syndrome characterized by variable degrees of limb deficiency (such as absent radius, ulna or thumb), hypoglossia and sometimes micrognathia. It has been attributed to compression effects on the fetus and to time-sensitive interruptions in fetal blood perfusion. It has been associated with chorion villus sampling in the first trimester of pregnancy.

Osteochondromatosis

See Ollier syndrome

Osteogenesis imperfecta

Osteogenesis imperfecta occurs in four different types.

Type I is an autosomal dominant disorder in which there appears to be a quantitative defect in the production of procollagen type I. It is characterized by short stature, often short limbs, fragile bones, biconcave vertebral flattening, blue sclera, thin skin and sclera, hyperextensibility and sometimes dislocation of joints, inguinal and umbilical hernias, capillary fragility with bleeding, and otosclerosis and deafness in adult life.

Type II may be due to sporadic mutation of an autosomal dominant gene, but in some cases it is an autosomal recessive disorder. It is characterized by prenatal growth deficiency, short limbs, short and broad long bones, poorly mineralized long bones, multiple fractures, blue sclera, and sometimes hydrocephalus. The child is stillborn or dies in early infancy.

Type III is a mosaic condition characterized by short stature, angulation and bowing of limbs, likelihood of multiple fractures, and normal sclera.

Type IV is an autosomal dominant disorder characterized by osteoporosis, likelihood of fractures, slight deformity of long bones, and normal sclera.

Osteohypertrophic angioectases
See Klippel–Trenaunay–Weber syndrome

Osteopetrosis, autosomal recessive–lethal

Autosomal recessive–lethal osteopetrosis is a severe osteopetrosis in which bones are dense, thick and fragile, with compression of bone marrow and cranial nerves, and hydrocephalus. Levels of alkaline phosphatase and serum phosphorus are raised, and serum calcium is likely to be low. It may be due to an abnormality of thyrocalcitonin metabolism. Death occurs in childhood or adolescence from infection, anemia, or bleeding.

Oto–palato–digital syndrome type I
See Taybi syndrome

Oto–palato–digital syndrome type II

Oto–palato–digital syndrome type II is an X-linked condition characterized by conductive hearing loss, cleft palate, hypertelorism, small mouth, micrognathia, polydactyly, syndactyly, flexed overlapping fingers, small or absent fibulae, and, sometimes, mental retardation. Death in infancy is common.

Ovarian cyst

Ovarian cyst occurs rarely in the neonate. It presents as an abdominal mass which can fill the abdomen, rupture or develop torsion.

P

Pachyonychia congenita

Pachyonychia congenita is an autosomal dominant disorder characterized by thick nails, hyperkeratosis of the palms and soles, leukoplakia of the mucous membrane of the mouth and tongue, and eruption of some teeth before birth.

Pagon syndrome
See CHARGE syndrome

Pallister syndrome

Other name Killian/Teschler–Nicola syndrome

Pallister syndrome is characterized by severe mental retardation, upslanting palpebral fissures, sparse eyebrows and eyelashes, hypertelorism, prominent forehead, strabismus, protruding lower lip, broad hands, short fingers, and, sometimes, microcephaly, macroglossia, hypermobile joints, and congenital dislocation of the hips. Tetrasomy 12p, total or mosaic, is present in skin fibroblasts, but not in peripheral blood.

Pallister–Hall syndrome

Pallister–Hall syndrome is characterized by a hamartoblastoma on the inferior surface of the cerebrum, hypopituitarism, endocardial cushion defects, hypoplasia or absence of the epiglottis, absence or abnormal lobulation of a lung, syndactyly and other deformities of the fingers and toes, rectal atresia, and imperforate anus. Other features can be cleft lip and palate, microphthalmia, hemivertebrae, fused ribs, congenital dislocation of the hip, and pancreatic hypoplasia.

Pallotta syndrome

Pallotta syndrome is a congenital syndrome characterized by coloboma of the iris, epicanthic folds, hypertelorism, and mental and motor retardation.

Pancreatic agenesis

Pancreatic agenesis in the infant can cause diabetes mellitus, edema, steatorrhea, hypoproteinemia, and a failure to thrive.

Pancreatic annulus

Annular pancreas is a ring of pancreas embracing the duodenum. It is due to persistence and growth of the dorsal pancreatic bud, which grows round the pancreas to unite with the ventral pancreatic bulb. Partial obstruction can occur, with abdominal distension and vomiting. Associated conditions can be Down syndrome, intestinal malrotation, duodenal atresia, and duodenal stenosis.

Papillon–Psaume syndrome

Papillon–Psaume syndrome is an autosomal dominant condition characterized by microcephaly, malformed canthi of the eye, defective alar cartilage of the nose, webbed fingers, tremor, frontal alopecia, defects of lip and palate, with normal or below-normal growth. It is lethal to males; only females survive.

Parachute mitral valve syndrome

See Shone syndrome

Parry–Romberg syndrome

Other name Facial hemiatrophy

Parry–Romberg syndrome is a progressive wasting of some or all of the tissues on one side of the face and sometimes beyond the face. The cause is unknown. It can be congenital, but it usually begins during the second decade. The wasting involves all the tissues of the face - skin, subcutaneous tissues, connective tissue, muscle, cartilage, and bone. The tongue, soft palate, larynx, and external ear can be affected. There may be atrophy of the cerebral hemisphere on the affected side. The atrophy can involve the neck, and, rarely, the breast. Very rarely, both sides of the face are affected. Associated conditions can be epileptic seizures, migraine, neuralgic facial pain, sensory impairment, vitiligo and syringomyelia.

Partial thoracic stomach

See Esophageal shortening

Partial trisomy 10q syndrome

Partial trisomy 10q syndrome is characterized by growth deficiency of prenatal origin, microcephaly, abnormal facies, cleft palate, heart, renal, ocular and cerebral anomalies, severe mental retardation, and other anomalies, with about one half of the patients dying within the first year of life.

Patau syndrome

Other name Trisomy 13 syndrome

Patau syndrome is characterized by multiple abnormalities, including scalp defects, coloboma, hypertelorism, cleft palate, deformed ears, congenital heart disease, an abnormal thumb, hydronephrosis, hydroureter, bicornuate uterus, and mental retardation. Death usually occurs in the first year of life.

Patent ductus arteriosus

The ductus arteriosus normally closes within 10–15 h after birth and the onset of respiration, with permanent structural changes taking up to 3 weeks. It becomes functionally closed when the pulmonary vascular pressure drops to a level lower than the systemic vascular pressure. Oxygen plays a part in constricting it. Failure to close is common in preterm infants; maternal rubella can be a factor. The female : male ratio is 2 : 1. Patent ductus arteriosus is the commonest form of aortopulmonary circulation. It results in an increased flow of blood through the left atrium and ventricle and also through the aorta and pulmonary artery. The size of the ductus varies, with its usual diameter 0.5–0.7 cm. Aneurysmal dilatation can occur. Patent ductus arteriosus can occur as an isolated anomaly or be associated with other anomalies, usually ventricular septal defect or coarctation of the aorta. Eighty percent of preterm infants have a duct that remains patent for the first four postnatal days, but only one-third have a shunt large enough to cause symptoms.

Patent urachus

Patent urachus is a failure of the urachus to become obliterated with the discharge of urine from the bladder through the umbilicus.

Pearson syndrome

Pearson syndrome is a disorder of mitochondrial inheritance and is characterized by lactic acidosis, pancytopenia and pancreatic insufficiency.

Pectoral muscle deficiency

Congenital deficiency of the pectoral muscles can occur on one side. It can be associated with hypoplasia of the breast and abnormalities of ribs 2–4. It can be a feature of Poland syndrome.

Pectus carinatum

Other name Pigeon chest

Pectus carinatum is a congenital forward projection of the sternum, usually with recession of the ribs. It is usually symptomless.

Pectus excavatum

Other name Tunnel chest

Pectus excavatum is a congenital abnormality of the front of the chest in which, below a normal manubrium, the sternum is depressed together with the anterior parts of the attached ribs, with the production of a concavity that is at its maximum at the xiphosternal junction. The depression is slight at birth and increases later. The cause is unknown; it has been attributed to respiratory obstruction, abnormal action of pectoral muscles or the diaphragm, and abnormal growth of sternal cartilage.

PEHO syndrome

PEHO syndrome is a progressive infantile encephalopathy characterized by:
PE – progressive encephalopathy
H – hypsarrhythmia
O – optic atrophy
Other features can be puffiness or edema of the extremities, spasms, and severe mental retardation.

Pena-Shokeir syndrome

Other name Fetal akinesia/hypokinesia sequence

Pena-Shokeir syndrome is an autosomal recessive condition in about half the cases. Decreased movements are observed *in utero* and there is impaired fetal growth. The umbilical cord may be unusually short. Premature birth can occur and about 30% are stillborn. The principal feature is ankyloses of elbows, knees, hips and ankles. Other features are hypertelorism, imperfect development of the mandible, cryptorchidism, and pulmonary hypoplasia, the last being a common cause of death within the first month of life.

Penile deformities

The penis may be unsually small (micropenis), absent, duplicated, webbed or concealed. Absence of the penis can be associated with cryptorchidism, inguinal hernia, hydrocele, anal stricture, imperforate anus, rectovesical fistula, and renal agenesis.

Penta X syndrome
See XXXXX syndrome

Perheentupa syndrome

Other name Mulibrey-nanism syndrome

Perheentupa syndrome is an autososmal recessive condition characterized by:
MU – muscle abnormalities
LI – liver abnormalities
BR – brain abnormalities
EY – eye abnormalities
nanism – dwarfism
Features are muscle fibroplasia and hypotonia, hepatomegaly, prenatal growth deficiency, relatively large hands and feet, dolicocephaly, triangular face, retinal pigment abnormalities, and constrictive pericarditis. The intelligence is within the normal range.

Pericardial cyst

Cyst of the pericardium is rare. The most common site is the right costophrenic angle. It is usually unilocular and filled with clear fluid. It is usually symptomless; torsion of the cyst can cause chest pain.

Pericardial defect

Pericardial defect is rare. The male : female ratio is 3 : 1. The most common form is a partial defect of the left pericardium. The defect may be familial. It is due to a defect either in the formation of the pleuropericardial membrane or, if diaphragmatic, of the septum transversum. Clinical features can be chest pain or discomfort and palpitations. Strangulation of the heart between the diaphragm and the pulmonary ligament has occurred in total absence of the pericardium. Associated features are common and include bicuspid aortic valve, atrial septal defect, bronchogenic cyts, and pulmonary sequestration.

Persistent pulmonary hypertension of the newborn

Persistent pulmonary hypertension of the newborn is characterized by suprasystemic pulmonary arterial pressure and right-to-left shunting of blood through the foramen ovale and ductus arteriosus. Affected infants are likely to develop respiratory distress and cyanosis within 12 h of birth. About 20–40% are likely to die; survivors may have some neurological impairment.

Peter-plus syndrome

Peter-plus syndrome is a congenital disorder characterized by the Peter anomaly (anterior ocular chamber cleavage anomaly), sclerocornea, brachycephaly, and short stature. The facies is similar to that of Robinow syndrome. Other features can be cleft lip and palate, cardiovascular anomalies, mental retardation and developmental delay.

Pfeiffer acrocephalosyndactyly syndrome

Pfeiffer acrocephalosyndactyly syndrome is characterized by craniosynostosis, acrocephaly, soft-tissue syndactyly, and broad deviated thumbs.

Pfeiffer brachycephaly syndrome

Pfeiffer brachycephaly syndrome is an autosomal dominant condition characterized by brachycephaly with a cloverleaf configuration, hydrocephaly, hypertelorism, beaked nose, high-arched palate, choanal atresia, broad thumbs and big toes, and, sometimes, congenital pyloric stenosis and anal malposition.

Pharyngeal diverticula

Congenital lateral pharyngeal diverticula are very rare. They are usually unilateral. Most arise from the second branchial cleft, with the track passing between the internal and external carotid arteries to open into the pharynx. They can arise from the third and fourth clefts. The patient presents with recurrent infected swellings in the neck.

Congenital posterior pharyngeal diverticula are very rare. They arise from above the cricopharyngeal muscle and are lined by normal pharyngeal mucosa. They can present in the neonatal period with symptoms similar to those of esophageal atresia.

Phenylketonuria

Phenylketonuria is an autosomal recessive condition and an inborn error of amino acid metabolism. The incidence is about 1 in 12 000, but there are considerable racial differences; the frequency in the Japanese is less than 1 in 200 000. There is an almost total absence of phenylalanine hydroxylase activity, an inability to convert phenylalanine into tyrosine, and an accumulation of phenylalanine in the tissues, blood, and urine. Neonates usually appear normal, but if the condition is not treated, brain damage causes mental retardation and neurological abnormalities.

Piebaldism

Piebaldism is an autosomal dominant condition of patchy amelanotic areas of skin. A white forelock can be a feature. Other features can be sensorineural deafness and mental retardation.

Pierre Robin syndrome

Other name First and second arch syndrome

Pierre Robin syndrome is an autosomal dominant condition characterized by multiple abnormalities, including a hypoplastic mandible and receding chin, cataract, sensorineural deafness, posterior displacement of the tongue (which obstructs breathing and can be an anesthesiological hazard), cleft soft and hard palate without cleft of the chin, a small epiglottis, and abnormalities of the fingers and toes. Intelligence may be normal or low. The gag reflex can be absent and attacks of choking and cyanosis can occur.

See also Catel–Manzke syndrome

Pigeon chest
See Pectus carinatum

Poland syndrome

Poland syndrome is a group of unilateral congenital anomalies of the chest wall with or without involvement of the arm on the same side. The right side is affected twice as often as the left side and there is a 3:1 male:female predominance. The commonest abnormality is absence of the pectoralis major and minor muscles. Syndactyly with absence of the sternal head of the pectoralis major can occur. The syndrome is thought not to be of genetic origin and may have a vascular cause.

Polycystic kidney disease

Polycystic kidney disease can be autosomal dominant or autosomal recessive.

Autosomal dominant polycystic kidney disease
Autosomal dominant polycystic kidney disease usually presents in adult life, but it can occur in the fetus and the newborn. Most of the cysts do not arise in the tubules and their origin is uncertain; those that do arise in the tubules are globular and can arise in any part of the tubule. The neonate may be symptom-free or present with a large cystic mass, and develop hypertension and renal failure. The infant may be stillborn or die within a few days. It is suggested that the condition is a systemic disorder due to a defect in the synthesis of extracellular matrix, and the responsible gene has been located on the short arm of chromosome 16. Associated conditions are colonic diverticula, mitral valve prolapse, incompetence of the mitral, tricuspid, and aortic valves, cerebral aneurysms, and hepatic and pancreatic cysts.

Autosomal recessive polycystic kidney disease
Autosomal recessive polycystic kidney disease shows multiple cysts arising in the renal tubules. The neonate presents with an enlarged abdomen and progressively enlarging kidneys. A few patients have normal or near-normal renal function, but most show polyuria, hypertension, failure to thrive, and renal failure. Associated conditions are hepatic fibrosis and bile duct hyperplasia and dilatation.

Polydactyly

Polydactyly is an autosomal dominant condition, with incomplete penetrance, especially common in African people. Disorders in which polydactyly is a feature include Bardet–Biedl syndrome, Ellis–van Creveld syndrome, Jeune syndrome, and trisomy 13.

Polymicrogyria

Polymicrogyria is a congenital abnormality of the cerebral cortex in which the gyri are thin and set in an abnormal pattern. Other abnormalities of the brain may be present. The condition can be due to damage *in utero* by several genetic, ischemic, and biochemical conditions.

Polyostotic fibrous dysplasia
See Albright syndrome

Pompe syndrome
See Glycogen storage disease II

Popliteal web syndrome

Popliteal web syndrome is an autosomal dominant condition characterized by popliteal and other webs, cleft lip with or without cleft palate, syndactyly, absent or defective teeth, absent eyebrows and lashes, sparse, brittle, short scalp hair, toe-nail dysplasia, cryptorchidism, scrotal dysplasia, or hypoplasia of the labia majora.

Polysplenia syndrome

Polysplenia syndrome is characterized by multiple small spleens in the right and left sides of the abdomen and occasionally in the midline. Associated conditions can be transposition of the liver and spleen, malrotation of the bowel, absence of the gallbladder, dextrocardia, congenital heart disease, abnormalities of the great veins, and bilateral bilobed lungs.

Postaxial acrofacial dysostosis syndrome

Other name Miller syndrome

Postaxial acrofacial dysostosis syndrome is an autosomal recessive condition in which there can be limb deficiencies most severe on the postaxial side (the medial aspect of the upper arm and the lateral aspect of the lower leg), malar hypoplasia, colobomas of the eyelid, ectropion, micrognathia, cleft lip and palate, and abnormally shaped ears. Congenital heart disease and conductive hearing loss are sometimes present. The intelligence is usually normal.

Potter syndrome

Potter syndrome is characterized by bilateral renal agenesis, pulmonary hypoplasia, skeletal abnormalities, gastrointestinal malformations, and a typical 'Potter facies' – a parrot-shaped nose, wide-set eyes, low-set ears, a fold of skin extending from the medial canthus to the cheek, and a receding chin. With absence of the kidneys, death in the first few days of life is inevitable.

Prader–Willi syndrome

Prader–Willi syndrome is a relatively common congenital disorder with an incidence of about 1 in 10 000 live births. There is a paternal microdeletion involving chromosome 15q. It is characterized by weak intrauterine movements, breech presentation, hypotonia, delayed attainment of developmental milestones, small hands and feet, small genitalia, undescended testes, almond-shaped eyes, possible cardiovascular abnormalities, overeating and stealing of food, body temperature variations, and mental retardation. Obstructive sleep apnea due to hypertrophy of the tonsils can occur. Diabetes mellitus can be an association.

Pre-auricular sinus
See External ear disorders

Primary atelectasis
See Immature lung syndrome

Primordial small stature with macrocrania

Primordial small stature with macrocrania is a condition of uncertain etiology and is characterized by small stature, large dolicocephalic head, dysmorphic facies, blepharophimosis, hypogonadism and cryptorchidism.

Proboscis lateralis

Proboscis lateralis is a very rare appendage about 2 cm long, arising from the region of the inner canthus. It is soft and freely movable, with an orifice at the tip. It may represent the nasolacrimal duct. Absent cribriform plate and imperforate anterior naris can be associated conditions.

Progeria

See Hutchinson–Gilford syndrome

Progressive arthro-ophthalmopathy

See Stickler syndrome

Prolapsed mitral valve syndrome

Other name Barlow syndrome

Prolapsed mitral valve syndrome is a form of congenital heart disease in which one or both leaflets of the mitral valve protrude into the left atrium during the systolic phase of ventricular contraction. It is probably the commonest form of congenital heart disease, as echocardiography has shown that it is present in 10–15% of the general population. It can be familial and there is a female : male ratio of 2 : 1. The mitral valve is affected with a myxomatous degeneration of unknown causation. Clinical features include chest pain, usually sharp and limited to the left side of the chest (which makes it liable to be thought to be angina pectoris due to coronary insufficiency), cardiac arrhythmias of various kinds, and, sometimes, complete atrioventricular block. The characteristic physical findings are a high-pitched systolic click and a late systolic or pansystolic murmur. The average lifespan can be unaffected, but it is reduced by severe mitral regurgitation, severe cardiac arrhythmias, or bacterial endocarditis. Sudden death is rare.

See also Heart malformations

Propionic acidemia

Propionic acidemia is an autosomal recessive condition in which there is a metabolic defect at the distal segment of the isoleucine and valine degradative pathways. Prenatal diagnosis is available. Clinical features are severe neonatal acidosis, lethargy, poor feeding, rapid respiration, vomiting, and, without adequate treatment, coma and death in the neonatal period. Survivors can have mental retardation, infections, failure to thrive, and recurrent attacks of acidosis, with death in early childhood.

Proteus syndrome

Proteus syndrome is a congenital syndrome characterized by thickening of the skin and subcutaneous tissues, subcutaneous masses, vascular disorders, epidermal nevi, and macrodactyly. Other features can be unilateral gigantism, bony prominences of the skull, scoliosis or kyphosis, muscle atrophy, and convulsions.

Prune belly syndrome

Other name Eagle–Barrett syndrome

In prune belly syndrome there is a congenital absence of the muscles of the anterior abdominal wall, and the lax excessive skin of the abdomen looks like the wrinkled skin of a prune. Associated conditions are urethral obstruction, an enlarged bladder, enlarged ureters, undescended testes, pulmonary hypoplasia, and lower limb arthrogryposis (flexion contractures), the last probably due to oligohydramnios. The male : female ratio is 2 : 1. It can occur spasmodically, as an X-linked transmission, associated with chromosomal abnormalities, and as a familial occurrence, associated with congenital deafness and mental retardation. Affected girls show only absence of the abdominal muscles. About 20% are stillborn or die within the first 4 weeks of life; 50% die within 2 years. Diagnosis can be made *in utero* by ultrasound by 21 weeks gestation.

Pseudo-Hurler polydystrophy syndrome

Other name Mucolipoidosis III

Pseudo-Hurler polydystrophy syndrome appears as a mild variety of Hurler syndrome without enlargement of the liver. At birth, the only features may be aortic valve disease and inguinal hernia, and in the first few years of life, the features become coarse, growth is deficient, joints become stiff, slight corneal opacities can develop, central nervous function deteriorates, and a mild degree of mental retardation is found on testing.

Ptosis

Congenital ptosis is a congenital inability to raise one or both upper eyelids. It may be a solitary defect or it may be associated with an inability to rotate the eye upwards. As an isolated defect, it is usually transmitted as a dominant trait. There is an incomplete development of the superior rectus and levator palpebrae muscles. It can occur intermittently on one side as a synkinetic phenomenon with each movement of the jaw in Marcus Gunn jaw-winking condition.

Pulmonary agenesis

Unilateral pulmonary agenesis is absence of one lung. It can be associated with congenital abnormalities of the heart, gastrointestinal tract, vertebrae, genitourinary tract (especially absence of a kidney), and ipsilateral limbs. Right pulmonary agenesis can be fatal in infancy. The single lung can be normal or have developmental anomalies. Bilateral agenesis can be associated with anencephaly, cardiovascular malformations, and absence of the spleen. It is incompatible with extrauterine life.

Pulmonary aplasia

Bilateral aplasia (imperfect development) of the lungs can be primary or secondary. Primary aplasia is of unknown origin. Secondary aplasia is more common and is associated with pulmonary vascular anomalies, pleural effusion, diaphragmatic hernia, bilateral renal agenesis, and prolonged leakage of amniotic fluid. It can be a feature of thanatophoric dysplasia. Clinical features are likely to be respiratory distress and cyanosis.

Pulmonary arteriovenous fistula

Pulmonary arteriovenous fistula can be single or multiple and very variable in size. It can cause neonatal cyanosis, and if it is large, it can cause respiratory difficulties.

Pulmonary atresia with intact ventricular membrane

In pulmonary atresia with intact ventricular membrane, the pulmonary valve is an imperforate membrane, the right ventricle is hypoplastic, sometimes having a volume at birth of only 1–2 ml, and the annulus of the tricuspid valve is hypoplastic and its chordae fused together, making the valve stenotic. The right ventricle is enlarged and its wall hypertrophic. The pulmonary arteries are normal. The incidence is 1 in 14 000 live births.

See also Heart malformations

Pulmonary cystic adenomatoid malformation

Pulmonary cystic adenomatoid malformation is a hamartomatous lesion with cysts, and affects any single lobe of a lung, greatly increasing its size, displacing the mediastinum, and impeding venous return to the heart. The cysts secrete fluid, communicate with airways, and, after birth, fill with air, compressing the lung still further. Stillbirth is common. Other congenital lesions can be present.

Pulmonary cystic adenomatoid malformation

Cystic adenomatoid malformation of the lung is a mass of cystic tissue in a lung. It appears to be due to an overgrowth of terminal bronchiolar tissue, and it may enlarge after birth due to a ball-valve communication with the airways. Associated conditions are hydrops fetalis, polyhydramnios, and hypoplasia of unaffected areas of the lung.

Pulmonary cysts

Congenital pulmonary cysts can be single or multiple; multiple cysts are always confined to one lung. They communicate with airways and are filled with air. A large single cyst or multiple cysts can cause dyspnea and tachypnea, and the heart may be shifted away from the affected side. A cyst can become infected.

Pulmonary hemangiomatosis

Pulmonary hemangiomatosis is a proliferation of small vessels in the lungs and airways. It can be part of a generalized hemangiomatosis involving other organs. Clinical features can be dyspnea and clubbing of the fingers. Many cases are symptomless. Hemoptysis can occur and bleeding can be a cause of death.

Pulmonary hypertension

Congenital pulmonary hypertension is a rare condition, and is due to obstruction of the pulmonary blood flow in the pulmonary arteries.

Pulmonary hypoplasia

Pulmonary hypoplasia is defined as the condition in which the combined lung weight is less than 1.2% of body weight, the standardized autopsy lung volume is less than 60% of predicted lung volume, lung DNA is less than 100 mg/kg of body weight, or the radial alveolar count is less than 4. The infant has hypercapnia (excess of carbon dioxide in the blood) and can have pulmonary hypertension, and pneumothorax. The condition can be associated with lung compression by congenital diaphragmatic hernia, diaphragmatic eventration, pleural effusion, ascites, congenital thoracic dystrophy, and a large omphalocele. Associated conditions can be oligohydramnios, renal agenesis, renal dysplasia, and obstructive uropathy.

Pulmonary intralobular sequestration

Intralobular pulmonary sequestration is an embryonic cystic portion of a lung which receives its blood supply from the systemic circulation, usually from the aorta. It is thought to be due to a failure of normal pulmonary vascular development in fetal life, with a persistence of the blood supply to the embryonic lung from the dorsal aorta.

Pulmonary lobar emphysema

Congenital lobar emphysema of the lungs is overinflation of one lobe of a lung with respiratory distress. It has been attributed to bronchial cartilage deficiency, stenosis of the bronchial wall, and external pressure by an anomalous pulmonary artery. Congenital heart disease can be an associated condition.

Pulmonary lymphangiectasis

Congenital pulmonary lymphangiectasis is a congenital abnormality of pulmonary lymph vessels which are dilated with an excess of pleural fluid. The male : female ratio is 2 : 1. It can be associated with congenital heart diseases, and when it is, death in the neonatal period is likely. When it is not associated with congenital heart disease, it is likely to be asymptomatic, with survival into adult life.

Pulmonary sequestration

Pulmonary sequestration occurs when a lobe of the lung does not communicate with the tracheobronchial tree and derives its blood supply by anomalous arteries arising from the aorta above and below the diaphragm. The lobe is usually on the left side, with two-thirds of cases involving the left lower lobe. The condition is thought to be due to an accessory lung bud. There are usually no symptoms in the neonate. Associated congenital abnormalities can be congenital heart disease, diaphragmatic hernia, diaphragmatic eventration, and rib and vertebral abnormalities.

Pulmonary stenosis

Pulmonary stenosis is usually a stenosis of the pulmonary valve and not the pulmonary artery. The main pulmonary artery may be dilated above the stenosis. An early systolic ejection sound can be heard. Pulmonary hypertension can be present. The right ventricle can hypertrophy and develop signs of strain.

See also Heart malformations

Pulmonary stenosis with intact ventricular septum

In pulmonary stenosis with intact ventricular septum, the orifice of the pulmonary valve is narrowed by fusion of the three pulmonary commissures. The right ventricle is hypoplastic and, although small, is not as small as in pulmonary atresia with intact ventricular septum. The incidence is about 1 in 14 000 live births.

See also Heart malformations

Purine nucleoside phosphorylase deficiency

Purine nucleoside phosphorylase deficiency is a rare inherited disease characterized by severe T-cell immunodeficiency. Infants with this condition closely resemble infants with severe combined immunodeficiency. Clinical features include recurrent infections, developmental delay, neurological disorders (spasticity, tremor, ataxia, hypertonia, hypotonia), mental retardation, autoimmune hemolytic anemia, idiopathic thrombocytopenic purpura, and systemic lupus erythematosus. Death occurs in childhood or early adult life. The gene responsible has been assigned to chromosome 14.

Pyknodysostosis

Pyknodysostosis is characterized by small stature, osteosclerosis, frontal and occipital protuberances, delayed closure of fontanels, dysplasia of distal phalanges, and a liability to have multiple fractures.

Pyle syndrome

Pyle syndrome is an autosomal condition and a form of metaphyseal dysplasia, with slight supraorbital hyperplasia, thickening of the calcarium, ribs, pubic, and ischial bones, limited elbow extension, and genu valgum.

Pyruvic acidemia

Pyruvic acidemia is due to a defect in pyruvate oxidation. Clinical features develop in the neonatal period with metabolic acidosis, lethargy, hypotonia, and rapid respirations. The blood levels of pyruvate and lactate are increased. Death can occur in early childhood; survivors can have permanent neurological damage.

R

Rabenhorst syndrome

Rabenhorst syndrome is probably an autosomal dominant disorder. It is characterized by asthenic physique, facial dysmorphism with a thin nose, mongoloid slant of the palpebral fissures and adherent ear lobules, a high palate, ventricular septal defect, pulmonary valve stenosis, and syndactyly of toes 2 and 3.

Raer syndrome

See Townes syndrome

Rapp–Hodgkin ectodermal dysplasia syndrome

Rapp–Hodgkin ectodermal dysplasia syndrome is a very rare autosomal dominant disorder characterized by growth deficiency, diminished sweat secretion and, in consequence, hyperthermia, poor teeth development, and, sometimes, cleft lip, cleft palate, or cleft uvula.

Recklinghausen syndrome

Other name Neurofibromatosis

Recklinghausen syndrome is an autosomal dominant disorder with high penetrance and wide variability of expression. It is characterized by:

(1) Multiple neurofibromas on nerve trunks, nerve plexuses, cranial and spinal nerves; sarcomatous changes can develop in these neurofibromas;

(2) Café-au-lait spots or larger pigmented areas in the skin; and

(3) Sessile or pedunculated polyps and swellings of the skin. An acoustic neurofibroma can cause deafness, facial weakness and anesthesia in the distribution of the trigeminal nerve on the same side. A neurofibroma within the orbit can cause proptosis and optic failure. An optic nerve glioma is an association; it is slow-growing and most likely to occur in childhood.

Rectal agenesis

Agenesis of the rectum is a failure of development of the rectum. There may be a rectal fistula through which meconium can be passed. Males may have agenesis with or without a fistula, which, if present, can open rectourethrally or rectovesically. In females, a fistula is likely to open into the vagina or into the urogenital sinus (the passageway for both vagina and urethra).

Rectal atresia

Atresia of the rectum is due to a congenital membrane which obstructs the rectum just above the levator sling. The clinical feature is a failure to pass meconium.

Reifenstein syndrome

Reifenstein syndrome is similar to Klinefelter syndrome but the XY-chromosome pattern is normal. Clinical features are gynecomastia and a mild degree of feminization. The testes and androgen levels are near normal.

Renal agenesis

Renal agenesis can be unilateral or bilateral.

Unilateral agenesis

Renal agenesis has an incidence of 1 in 1100 births, with a male : female ratio of 8 : 1. It can be an autosomal dominant condition in some females. It is more common on the left side than the right. It can be compatible with longevity. Associated conditions can be ipsilateral absence or maldevelopment of the ureter, ipsilateral agenesis of the adrenal gland, and genital abnormalities. In the female, there can be double or septate uterus and maldevelopment of the vagina. There can also be cardiac, gastrointestinal, and musculoskeletal anomalies. Associated conditions are VATER syndrome, Turner syndrome and Poland syndrome.

Bilateral agenesis

In bilateral agenesis, the kidneys are completely absent or represented by a small mass of tissue containing primitive glomerular elements. The condition is rare, with a reported incidence varying from 1 in 4800 to 1 in 10 000. It can be an autosomal recessive condition. Prenatal ultrasonic screening shows absence of kidneys and severe oligohydramnios. About 40% of those affected are stillborn; the others die usually within 48 hours of birth. Associated conditions are absence of the ureters, hypoplastic bladder, absent renal artery, undescended or agenetic testes, facial abnormalities ('Potter face'), and abnormal development of the legs.

Renal dysplasia

Renal dysplasia is an abnormal development of renal tissue in which the glomeruli and tubules are defective and enclosed in fibrous tissue. The kidneys contain many cysts and are grossly malformed. Associated conditions are ureteric obstructive abnormalities, hydronephrosis, and prune belly syndrome.

Renal ectopia

Renal ectopia is the presence of a kidney in an abnormal position, usually the pelvis, and less commonly in the lumbar region of the thorax. An ectopic kidney may be symptomless, but it is liable to injury if it is situated in a less protected area than a normally placed kidney. It can present as an abdominal mass. It may function poorly. Associated conditions can be a renal fusion abnormality and vesicoureteral reflux.

A *crossed fused renal ectopia* occurs when one kidney is present in the opposite side of the body and is fused to the other kidney. It occurs in about 1 in 1000 live births, and the male : female ratio is 2 : 1. Usually, the left kidney has crossed to the right side and fused with the right kidney, which lies superior to it, with its lower pole fused with the upper pole of the kidney beneath. The condition may be symptomless, or present as an abdominal mass. Associated conditions can be vesicoureteral reflux and hydronephrosis.

Renal hypoplasia

Renal hypoplasia is a congenital deficiency of normal renal tissue. It is usually bilateral and may be insufficient to maintain normal growth. It can occur in the fetal alcohol syndrome. Two forms are described: segmental hypoplasia and oligomeganephronia. *Segmental hypoplasia* may be the result of pyelonephritis and scarring and not a true congenital abnormality; it can be bilateral or unilateral, and causes hypertension. *Oligomeganephronia* is a bilateral condition in which the number of nephrons is greatly reduced and those that are present are hypertrophied. The male : female incidence is 3 : 1. In the neonatal period and early infancy, the condition can be asymptomatic or there may be dehydration, fever, vomiting, proteinuria, tubular dysfunction with polyuria, polydipsia and acidosis. Renal insufficiency can occur in the neonatal period or infancy, but the condition can become stable. Growth is usually poor. Renal failure usually develops at 5–15 years.

Renal tubular acidosis

See Fanconi syndrome

Retinal dystrophia

Congenital retinal dystrophia is a condition in which dysfunction of retinal receptors causes severe visual impairment from early infancy. Most causes are autosomal recessive conditions. The retina appears to be normal or near normal. The electroretinogram is absent or severely attenuated. Visual evoked responses are usually reduced. Clinical conditions include Leber congenital amaurosis, Joubert syndrome and Zellweger syndrome.

Retinopathy of prematurity

Other name Retrolental fibroplasia

Retinopathy of prematurity is due to the administration of high oxygen concentrations to premature infants, with the development of vasoconstriction of retinal vessels, occlusion of the vessels, fibrous proliferation, and blindness developing within a few weeks.

Retrolental fibroplasia

See Retinopathy of prematurity

Rhizomelic chondrodysplasia punctata syndrome

Rhizomelic chondrodysplasia punctata syndrome is an autosomal recessive condition characterized by punctate chondrodystrophy, microcephaly, cataracts, multiple joint contractures, respiratory insufficiency, and mental retardation. Most infants die in the postnatal period.

Rieger syndrome

Rieger syndrome is a genetically determined syndrome, most frequent as a dominant condition, but sporadic cases are seen and this suggests a recessive pattern also. It is characterized by a posterior embryotoxon (an opaque ring at the margin of the cornea), a prominent Schwalbe line (the peripheral edge of the Descemet membrane), adhesions of the iris to the Schwalbe line, and glaucoma. Other features can be hypertelorism, hypoplasia of the malar bones, congenital absence of some teeth, and mental retardation.

Ring chromosome 13

The clinical features associated with ring chromosome 13 are anencephaly, cranial vault defects, hypertelorism, hypoplasia of the adrenal glands, hypoplasia of the gallbladder, and imperforate anus. The infant dies shortly after birth.

Ritscher–Schinzel syndrome
See C3 syndrome

Robert syndrome

Robert syndrome is an autosomal recessive condition characterized by prenatal growth deficiency, limb abnormalities (varying from phocomelia of all limbs to radial hypoplasia), mental retardation, and, sometimes, cleft lip and palate.

Robinow syndrome

Other name Fetal face syndrome

Robinow syndrome is an autosomal dominant disorder characterized by macrocephaly, large anterior fontanel, frontal bossing, triangular mouth with down-turned corners, short forearms, brachydactyly, hemivertebrae, cryptorchidism, and small external genitalia.

Rokitansky syndrome

Rokitansky syndrome is the result of a defect in the development of the caudal paramesonephric duct. The uterus is rudimentary or bicornuate and the upper end of the vagina is absent; the lower end is present as a blind pouch. The patient does not menstruate. The ovaries, Fallopian tubes, and secondary sexual characteristics are normal. Other defects in structures derived from the mesonephric ridge can produce renal agenesis or hypoplasia and duplication of the ureters. Other complications can be vertebral and rib abnormalities.

Rokitansky–Küster–Hauser syndrome
See Mayer–Rokitansky–Küster syndrome

Rubinstein–Taybi syndrome

Other name Broad thumb syndrome

Rubinstein–Taybi syndrome is characterized by multiple congenital abnormalities: microcephaly, abnormal facies (with a prominent forehead, a thin beaked nose, anti-mongoloid slant of the eyes), high-arched palate, low-set ears, cataracts, short stature, cardiac abnormalities, hirsutism, renal abnormalities, broad thumb and big toe, hemangiomas of the skin, cryptorchidism, a failure to thrive, and mental retardation. The chromosome assignment is 16p13.

Russell–Silver syndrome

Russell–Silver syndrome is an autosomal recessive condition characterized by physical growth retardation of prenatal origin, a small triangular face, abnormally curved fingers, webbed toes, café-au-lait spots on the skin, and mental retardation. Asymmetry of the body can be present, one side being larger than the other, and one leg longer than the other. Nephroblastoma can be a complication.

Ruvalcaba syndrome

Ruvalcaba syndrome is characterized by growth deficiency *in utero*, microcephaly, hypoplastic alae nasi, narrow maxilla, crowded teeth, small mouth, short limbs, short metacarpals, cryptorchidism, and mental retardation.

Ruvalcaba–Myhre–Smith syndrome

Ruvalcaba–Myhre–Smith syndrome is probably an autosomal dominant disorder. It is characterized by macrocephaly, ileal and colonic hamartomatous polyposis, and pigmented spots on the penis.

S

Sacral agenesis
See Caudal regression syndrome

Sacrococcygeal teratoma

Sacrococcygeal teratoma arises from the tip or inner surface of the coccyx and presents as a mass between the coccyx and rectum, or can be detected by rectal examination. The female : male incidence is 2–4 : 1. Of these teratomas, 60–70% are benign. Associated conditions are malformations of the hindgut, vertebrae, and genitourinary system.

Saethre–Chotzen syndrome

Other name Acrocephalosyndactyly type III

Saethre–Chotzen syndrome is an autosomal dominant condition characterized by acrocephaly that may be asymmetrical, partial syndactyly of digits 1–2 or 3–4, and failure of one or both testes. Other features can be hypertelorism, strabismus, low-set ears, a defect of the lacrimal ducts, highly-arched palate, mild hearing loss, and bending of the fingers medially or laterally.

Saldino–Noonan syndrome

Other name Short rib–polydactyly syndrome I

Saldino–Noonan syndrome is an autosomal recessive condition characterized by short limbs, a narrow chest, short ribs, polydactyly, anal atresia, renal and genital anomalies, and heart defects.

Sanfilippo syndrome

Other name Mucopolysaccharidosis III

Sanfilippo syndrome is an autosomal recessive disorder of mucopolysaccharide metabolism and is characterized by coarse features, joint stiffness, enlarged liver, and severe mental retardation. Death is common before 20 years of age. It can be due to a deficiency of heparan-N-sulfatase (type A), of N-acetyl-α-D-glucosaminidase (type B), of α-glucosaminidase (type C), or of N-acetyl-α-glucosaminide-6-sulfatase (type D). The biochemical forms are not clinically distinguished.

Scheie syndrome

Other name Mucopolysaccharidosis Is and V

Scheie syndrome is an autosomal recessive disorder characterized by mandibular prognathism, aortic valve defect, retinal pigmentation, inguinal and umbilical hernias, broad hands and feet, and the gradual development of joint limitation, hirsutism, and corneal clouding. There is an excess urinary excretion of dermatan sulfate.

Schinzel–Giedion syndrome

Schinzel–Giedion syndrome is probably an autosomal recessive condition. It is characterized by mid-face retraction, large patent fontanels and wide cranial sutures, a high protruding forehead, hypertelorism, abnormal ears, short forearms and legs, hypoplastic first ribs, hydronephrosis, ureteric distension, hypertrichosis, and severe mental retardation. Death is usual before 2 years of age.

Schizencephaly

Schizencephaly is a developmental cleft, bilateral or unilateral, in the cerebral mantle extending from the cortical surface to a ventricle. The brain, proximal to the cleft, may be normal, but that below is rudimentary and hypoplastic. The upper part of the cerebrum on both sides may be represented by a cyst covered with a paper-thin layer of nervous parenchyma. The diagnosis can be made by computerized tomography scan. Severely affected infants are likely to be severely mentally retarded and have spastic tetraplegia and fits.

Schmid–Fraccaro syndrome
See Cat-eye syndrome

Schwachman syndrome

Schwachman syndrome is an autosomal recessive disorder characterized by pancreatic insufficiency, reduced neutrophil chemotaxis, and metaphyseal dyschondroplasia. Clinical features include short stature, narrowing of the rib cage due to involvement of the ribs, musculoskeletal anomalies, recurrent infections, anemia, neutropenia, and thrombocytopenia.

Schwartz–Jampel syndrome

Other name Myotonic chondrodystrophy

Schwartz–Jampel syndrome is an autosomal myotonic dystrophy characterized by intrauterine growth deficiency, short stature, skeletal abnormalities, and an abnormal persistence of muscular contractions. Other features can be mental retardation, congenital dislocation of the hip, cataract, low hair line, low-set ears, and small testicles.

Scimitar syndrome

Scimitar syndrome is characterized by a hypoplastic right lung, systemic arterial blood supply to the right lung, dextrocardia, and anomalous right pulmonary venous drainage to the vena cava. It is so called because of its radiological appearance.

Sclerosteosis

Sclerosteosis is an autosomal recessive condition characterized by a progressive overgrowth and thickening of bone, slight or moderate gigantism, and syndactyly of the second and third fingers. Thickening of the skull can cause compression of foramina and hydrocephalus.

Seckel syndrome

Other name Bird-headed dwarfism

Seckel syndrome is an autosomal recessive condition characterized by short stature, a characteristic facies (microcephaly, large nose, abnormal ears, receding forehead, micrognathia), dislocation of the head of the radius, dislocation of the hip, trident hands, absence of some teeth, hypoplasia of the upper end of the fibula, 11 pairs of ribs, a reduction in the number of blood cells, cryptorchidism, and mental retardation.

Senger syndrome

Senger syndrome is a form of mitochondrial myopathy with bilateral congenital cataracts, hypotonia, cardiomyopathy, and intermittent attacks of lactic acidosis. The hypotonia and cataracts are present in the neonate; cardiomyopathy occurs in infancy. Sudden death can be due to a conduction defect of the heart.

Severe combined immunodeficiencies

Severe combined immunodeficiencies are a heterogeneous group of disorders characterized by a severe defect in T-cell differentiation or function. The frequency is 1 in 50 000–75 000 births. Maternal T cells are present in the infant's blood and can survive for months. In this condition, there may be no clinical features; when they are present, they are usually mild, with erythema, diarrhea, hepatitis, and eosinophilia. The thymus is seriously abnormal, with an absence of the lymphoid component and of Hassal's corpuscles, and defective differentiation of epithelial cells. Transfusion of non-irradiated blood products can cause a lethal graft-versus-host disease. Without a bone marrow transplantation, death within the first year of life is usual, but survival to over 2 years has been reported.

Mature T and B cells can be absent in 20–25% of patients with typical severe combined immunodeficiency, which is inherited as an autosomal recessive condition. Lymphopenia is present but is not total, as natural killer cells are present and functional.

Severe combined immunodeficiency can occur where there is an absence of immature and mature T cells with B cells present, often in increased number. This is inherited as an autosomal recessive or a recessive X-linked condition. The thymus is immature and without thymocytes.

Adenosine deaminase activity is defective in about 20% of cases of severe combined immunodeficiency. Clinical features include severe T and B lymphocytopenia, neurological disorders with dystonia and blindness of central origin, and with chondrodysostosis in about half the patients. The responsible gene is located on chromosome 20q13.4, and the degree of enzyme activity and immunodeficiency is determined by the various types of gene anomaly.

See also Omenn syndrome

Severe congenital sensorineural deafness
See Deaf mutism

Shapiro syndrome

Shapiro syndrome is characterized by agenesis of the corpus callosum and features of hypothalamic dysfunction, especially hypothermia.

Shokier syndrome

Shokier syndrome is an autosomal dominant condition characterized by congenital total permanent alopecia, psychomotor epilepsy, pyorrhea, and mental retardation.

Shone syndrome

Other name Parachute mitral valve syndrome

Shone syndrome consists of:

(1) A parachute deformity of the mitral valve, due to an insertion of all the chordae tendinae into a single pupillary muscle, with blood flow from the left atrium passing through the interchordal spaces, causing various degrees of functional mitral stenosis;

(2) A supravalvular mitral ring, an accumulation of connective tissue arising from the atrial surface of the mitral valve, with a reduction in the size of the mitral orifice;

(3) Valvular or subvalvular aortic stenosis; and

(4) Coarctation of the aorta.

Heart failure and pulmonary infections are complications.

Short-limb dwarfism with immunodeficiency

Short-limb dwarfism can be associated with immunodeficiency, varying from mild dysfunction to severe combined immunodeficiency. The condition is inherited as an autosomal recessive trait and can be present early in childhood or develop a few years later.

Short-rib syndrome

Short-rib syndrome is characterized by short ribs, short stature, short limbs, femoral bowing, cleft lip and palate, and severe respiratory failure. Polydactyly is not a feature.

Short rib–polydactyly syndrome I
See Saldino–Noonan syndrome

Short rib–polydactyly syndrome II
See Majewski syndrome

Short stature–joint dysplasia–erythema telangiectasia syndrome

Short stature–joint dysplasia–erythema telangiectasia is a syndrome of unknown causation. Clinical features are short stature, multiple symmetrical abnormalities of joints and bone, and, at about 2 years of age, the development of telangiectatic erythema on the face.

Shprintzen syndrome
See Velo–cardio–facial syndrome

Simpson–Golabi–Behmel syndrome

Simpson–Golabi–Behmel syndrome is characterized by prenatal postnatal overgrowth, coarse facial features, macrostomia, macroglossia, supernumerary nipples, finger-nail dysplasia, hypotonia, and cardiac conduction defects. Death can occur in the neonatal period.

Sirenomelia

Sirenomelia is a congenital condition in which the legs are fused together and there are no feet. The incidence is about 1 in 1 000 000 births. The maternal age may be markedly increased. Other congenital abnormalities are likely and may be neural tube defects, hydrocephalus, cleft lip and palate, esophageal atresia, septal defects of the heart, and defects of the radii.

Sjögren–Larsson syndrome

Sjögren–Larsson syndrome is an autosomal recessive disorder characterizeu by congenital ichthyosis of the skin, followed a year or two later by spastic weakness of the legs, retinitis pigmentosa, dysplasia of dental enamel, mental retardation, and, sometimes, epilepsy.

Sly syndrome

Other name Mucopolysaccharidosis VII

Sly syndrome is a form of mucopolysaccharidosis in which there is a deficiency of β-glucuronidase. It is characterized by coarse facies, corneal opacities, enlarged liver and spleen, umbilical hernia, inguinal hernia, aortic valve disease, pectum carinatum, and joint deformities.

Smith–Lemli–Opitz syndrome

Smith–Lemli–Opitz syndrome is an autosomal recessive condition characterized by multiple congenital abnormalities: microcephaly, a characteristic facies with micrognathia and anteverted nostrils, short stature, hypoplasia of the thymus, male genital abnormalities, syndactyly, and mental retardation. Cardiac, renal, and vertebral abnormalities may be present. The eyes may show strabismus, cataracts and ptosis. During the last 4 weeks of pregnancy, the maternal urinary estriol level is very low and sometimes unrecordable. The syndrome may be the result of a defect in fetal adrenal metabolism.

Smith–Magenis syndrome

Smith–Magenis syndrome shows an interstitial deletion of the short arm of chromosome 17 and is characterized by facial dysmorphism, brachycephaly, flat mid-face, short broad hands, mental retardation and behavioral problems.

Soloman syndrome
See Fuerstein–Mimms syndrome

Sotos syndrome

Other name Cerebral gigantism

Sotos syndrome is characterized by large body size for age in childhood, macrocephaly, frontal bossing, large jaw, hypertelorism, nystagmus, strabismus, clumsiness, developmental delay, moderate-to-severe mental retardation, and a higher risk than normal of developing tumors, especially hepatic tumors and Wilms tumor. In Japanese patients, congenital heart lesions and urogenital anomalies have been found.

Sphenoid sinus abnormalities

The sphenoid sinus may be absent or represented by a small air cell.

Spina bifida cystica

Spina bifida cystica is a failure of development of the vertebral laminae, most commonly in the lumbar region and associated with protrusion of the meninges and other contents of the spinal canal. It is a common abnormality, but the incidence has been declining over several years. The defect may be present at birth in several forms, with clinical features likely to be paralysis of the lower limb muscles, deformities of the feet, contraction of joints, absent sensation, and neurogenic bladder dysfunction, with variations varying with the site, size, and nature of the lesion.

A *meningocele* is a protrusion of meninges without any neural component, usually sited in the lumbar region, and usually covered by skin, but sometimes by a membrane that is liable to infection. Motor function in the legs is usually normal. A *meningomyelocele* is a herniated sac containing meninges and neural tissue. It is much more common than meningocele. The spinal cord above the lesion may be normal. *Lipomeningomyelocele* is a meningomyelocele overlain by a lipoma. A *syringomyelocele* is one in which the spinal cord shows hydromyelia (a dilatation of the central canal of the cord with an abnormal collection of fluid).

Microgyria of the brain can be present. Hydrocephalus is commonly an association of meningomyelocele.

Spina bifida occulta

Spina bifida occulta is a term used to describe (a) a severe spinal defect, usually of the lumbosacral spine, associated commonly with a pigmented or hairy patch of skin, and with the likelihood of neural tube defects in sibs and offspring; and (b) congenital absence of one or two vertebral arches, without clinical features, usually discovered incidentally on radiological examination of the spine for some condition, occurring in about 5% of the general population, and without risks to sibs and offspring.

Split hand
See Ectrodactyly

Spondylocostal dysostosis

Spondylocostal dysostosis is usually an autosomal recessive condition, occasionally autosomal dominant. It is characterized by a short trunk, barrel-shaped chest, spina bifida, and anomalies of ribs and vertebrae. Other features can be tetralogy of Fallot, pulmonary valve stenosis, renal and ureteric anomalies, syndactyly and club feet.

Spondyloepiphyseal dysplasia congenita

Spondyloepiphyseal dysplasia congenita is usually an autosomal dominant condition characterized by growth deficiency *in utero*, slowness of mineralization of epiphyses, short trunk, lumbar lordosis, hypoplasia of abdominal muscles, myopia, retinal detachment (50% of cases), hypotonia, and, sometimes, congenital dislocation of the hip.

Spondyloepiphyseal dysplasia tarda
See X-linked spondyloepiphyseal dysplasia tarda

Spondylometaphyseal dysplasia
See Kozlowski syndrome

Spondylothoracic dysplasia
See Jarcho–Levin syndrome

Stapes footplate fixation

Congenital fixation of the stapes footplate of the middle ear may be an isolated defect behind a normal tympanic plate; annular ligament is absent. Hearing is impaired, but does not become worse.

Steinert syndrome
See Myotonic dystrophy

Sternal abnormalities

Congenital abnormalities of the sternum can be:

(1) Pectus excavatum or carinatum;

(2) Upper sternal clefts (a failure of fusion in the upper part of the sternum); or

(3) A complete failure of fusion of the two halves of the sternum, which allows the heart and attached structures to protrude (ectopia cordis). Congenital abnormalities of the heart can be present.

Sternomastoid tumor

Sternomastoid tumor is a smooth hard oval mass in the sternomastoid muscle. It is composed of endomysial fibrosis with collagen and fibroblasts deposited around atrophying muscle fibers, and is therefore not a true tumor. Torticollis, rotation of the head to the opposite side, and facial and cranial asymmetry can be present. The lesion usually resolves within 12 months.

Stickler syndrome

Other name Progressive arthro-ophthalmopathy

Stickler syndrome is an autosomal dominant condition characterized by arthritis, cataracts, retinal detachment, and glaucoma. Other features can be tall stature, maxillary hypoplasia, flat facies, deafness, kyphoscoliosis, and cleft palate.

Strong syndrome

Strong syndrome is characterized by a familial right-sided aortic arch, asymmetrical abnormalities, and mental retardation.

Sturge–Weber syndrome

Sturge–Weber syndrome is characterized by capillary or cavernous hemangiomas within the cutaneous distribution of a branch of the trigeminal nerve on one side, associated with a predominantly venous hemangioma of the leptomeninges and cortical destruction below it. Complications are convulsions and hemiparesis.

Subglottic stenosis

Congenital subglottic stenosis is due to malformation of the cricoid cartilage. Mild degrees of stenosis can cause cough and hoarseness; severe obstruction causes stridor and respiratory distress.

Supernumerary kidney

A supernumerary kidney is a rare third kidney. It is small and has its own blood supply. It may be loosely attached to one of the other kidneys. The ureter may be bifid or duplicated, but there are usually no other abnormalities. Males and females are equally affected. In childhood, there are no symptoms, but in adult life, there may be attacks of pain and fever, hypertension, a palpable abdominal mass, and carcinoma, but in 25%, the additional kidney is asymptomatic.

Supraventricular tachycardia

Supraventricular tachycardia can be present with sudden severe cardiovascular collapse in the neonate, and it can be the cause of unexplained hydrops fetalis. It can present with tachypnea, pallor, and poor feeding. It can be intermittent.

Surdocardiac syndrome
See Jervell–Lange–Nielsen syndrome

Surviving twin syndrome

If one monozygotic twin should die *in utero*, emboli from the dead twin can enter the organs and tissues of the surviving twin and cause microinfarctions.

Sweaty foot syndrome
See Isovaleric acidemia

Symphalangism syndrome
See Multiple svnostosis svndrome

Syndactyly

Syndactyly, isolated and bilateral, occurs as an autosomal dominant condition. Disorders in which syndactyly is a feature include acrocephalosyndactyly, oral–facial–digital syndrome, and Poland syndrome.

Syndromatic bile duct paucity
See Alagille syndrome

Syringomyelocele
See Spina bifida cystica

T

TAR syndrome

TAR syndrome is an autosomal recessive condition in which there is an association of:
T – thrombocytopenia
AR – absence of the radius
Severe thrombocytopenia is present in infancy and usually decreases after 1 year of age. Many patients die in the first year of life from an intracranial hemorrhage.

Taussig–Bing syndrome

Taussig–Bing syndrome is a double-outlet right ventricle with transposition of the aorta. The aorta arises from the right ventricle and is slightly posterior to the pulmonary artery, which arises anteriorly from both ventricles. A sub-pulmonary ventricular septal defect is present.

Taybi syndrome

Other name Oto–palato–digital syndrome I

Taybi syndrome is characterized by conductive deafness, short stature, thick frontal bone and base of skull, cleft soft palate, teeth abnormalities, pectus excavatus, broad distal phalanges, short nails, and slight mental retardation.

T-cell receptor congenital immunodeficiencies

T-cell receptor congenital immunodeficiencies can be the cause of severe diarrhea, pneumonia, and failure to thrive, with death in infancy.

T–D–O syndrome
See Tricho–dento–osseous syndrome

Testis abnormalities

Except for maldescent (cryptorchidism), congenital abnormalities of the testis are rare. They can be:

(1) Agonadism: complete absence of both testes is rare. The chromosomal pattern is XY, which indicates that the testes must have been present in early fetal life and then absorbed. With bilateral agonadism, there is incomplete differentiation of the male genitalia. If there has been a gonadal failure before organization of the genital tract, the external genitalia will be female. If the failure has occurred during the period of male sex differentiation, ambiguous genitalia will be present. If the failure has occurred after the 16th week of gestation, the male genitalia will be established without testes, and the fetus develops as a male.

(2) Monorchidism: absence of one testis.

(3) Polyorchidism: more than two testes.

(4) Synorchidism: fusion of the testes, which occurs abdominally.

(5) Maldescent: *see* Cryptorchidism.

Tetrasomy 9p syndrome

Tetrasomy 9p syndrome appears to result from a translocation involving the chromosomal 9qh region. Clinical features are brachycephaly, hypertelorism, beaked nose, bilateral cleft lip and palate, low-set malformed ears, head defects, ambiguous genitalia, and severe mental retardation.

Thanatophoric dysplasia

Thanatophoric dysplasia (*thanatophoria* – death-bringing (Greek)) is a congenital disorder characterized by growth deficiency *in utero*, large cranium, low nasal bridge, short limbs, flat vertebrae, short ribs and narrow chest, and sometimes, brain abnormalities (microgyria, faulty organization in temporal lobe and cerebellum, absent corpus callosum), patent ductus arteriosus, auricular septal defect, horseshoe kidney, imperforate anus, hydronephrosis, and craniostenosis. The infant dies shortly after birth from respiratory insufficiency.

Third and fourth pharyngeal pouch syndrome
See DiGeorge syndrome

Thoracoschisis

Thoracoschisis is a congenital fissure in the chest wall.

Three-A syndrome

Three-A syndrome is characterized by:
adrenal insufficiency
absence of tears
achalasia of the cardia
Other features can be motor and sensory neuropathy, optic atrophy, ataxia, autonomic function impairment, and mental retardation.

Three-M syndrome

Three-M syndrome is named after the initial letter of the first authors (Miller, McKusick, Malvaux). It is a congenital and probably autosomal condition. It is characterized by low birth weight, short stature, dysmorphic features, hatchet-shaped face, relatively large head, prominent mouth and lips, short broad neck, prominent trapezius muscles, deformed sternum, slender ribs and long bones, prominent heels, and growth retardation. Spina bifida occulta may be present. Mental development is normal.

Thrombocytopenia with absence of radii

Thrombocytopenia (decreased production of platelets) can be associated with bilateral absence of the radii. The leukocyte count can be raised and include many immature forms.

Thyroid dysgenesis

Thyroid dysgenesis is a term used to describe absence or hypoplasia of the thyroid gland. It occurs in 1 in 4000 live births. The male : female ratio is 1 : 2. It is usually sporadic, but familial cases can occur. The infant usually appears normal at birth, with signs of hypothyroidism developing within a few weeks. There is an association with Down syndrome.

Thyrotoxicosis

Neonatal thyrotoxicosis is due to the transplacental passage of thyroid-stimulating antibody from a mother with thyrotoxicosis or Hashimoto thyroiditis. Clinical features are likely to be flushing, tachycardia, irritability, enlargement of the thyroid gland, exomphalos, cardiac arrhythmias, and poor weight gain. Cardiac failure and death can follow

Tietze syndrome

Tietze syndrome is a familial dominant condition in which albinism is associated with deafness and loss of the eyebrows.

Toe nail abnormalities

Big toe nails can be congenitally malaligned, and this can lead to thickened or ingrowing nails and inflammation, in later life.

Tongue tie
See Ankyloglossia inferior

Tonsil absence

Congenital absence of the palatine tonsil is a rare condition and is due to a defect of the second or third pharyngeal pouches. Associated conditions are congenital absence of the palatopharyngeal fold, microtia, and polydactyly.

Total anomalous pulmonary venous return

Total anomalous pulmonary venous return is a congenital malformation in which the pulmonary veins do not open into the right atrium but into the left atrium, usually by a single trunk. The abnormality is thought to be a failure of development of the common pulmonary vein, which normally connects the developing venous plexuses with the left atrium. Obstruction of the vein is present in varying degrees, with the presentation depending on the degree of obstruction. The incidence is about 1 in 17 000 live births. Clinical features are severe cyanosis, which does not respond to the administration of oxygen, rapid and difficult respiration, congestive heart failure, pulmonary venous congestion on chest radiograph, and right ventricular preponderance on an electrocardiogram.

See also Heart malformations

Townes–Brocks syndrome
See Townes syndrome

Townes syndrome

Other name Townes–Brocks syndrome; Raer syndrome

Townes syndrome is an autosomal dominant condition with variability in the severity of expression of individual features. It is characterized by anomalies of the ear, thumb, anus, and urinary system. The anomalies of the ears are imperfect development or enlargement. The anomalies of the thumb can be hypoplasia, three phalanges, or a supernumerary thumb. The anomalies of the anus can be imperforation, stenosis, or anterior displacement. Anomalies of the urinary system can be renal hypoplasia, urethral valves, and ureterovesical reflux.

Tracheal agenesis

Congenital agenesis of the trachea is usually associated with a bronchoesophageal fistula and commonly with malformations of the heart. It is incompatible with life after birth.

Tracheal stenosis

Tracheal stenosis is stenosis of a short or long segment of the trachea; the trachea and bronchi can be hypoplastic. Clinical features are stridor, wheezing and cyanotic episodes. Congenital malformations of other organs can be present.

Tracheobronchomalacia

Tracheobronchomalacia is a softness of the trachea and bronchi due to impaired development of their cartilages. During respiratory expiration the anterior and posterior walls of the trachea become approximated, with the production of wheezing and respiratory distress.

Tracheobronchomegaly

Other name Mounier–Kuhn syndrome

Tracheobronchomegaly is a congenital enlargement of the trachea and bronchi. The trachea can be 35–50 mm in diameter. The condition leads to attacks of bronchitis, bronchiolitis, pneumonia, emphysema, bronchiectasis, and pulmonary fibrosis. It may be associated with Ehlers–Danlos syndrome.

Tracheobronchopathia osteoplastica

Tracheobronchopathia osteoplastica is the presence of ectopic cartilage or bone between the cartilaginous rings of the trachea. Clinical features can be hoarseness, cough, respiratory difficulties, and, sometimes, hemoptysis.

Tracheoesophageal fistula

Tracheoesophageal fistula can occur on its own or as a part of ARTICLE-V syndrome (anal, renal, tracheal, intestinal, cardiac, limb, esophageal, and, sometimes, vertebral anomalies), of VATER syndrome (vertebral, anal, tracheoesophageal, renal, and radial anomalies), or of VACTEL syndrome (vertebral, anal, cardiac, tracheoesophageal, and limb anomalies). The incidence is 1 per 3000 live births. About 3% of infants are premature and 22% have a major cardiac malformation. The most common abnormality is an upper esophageal pouch with a fistulous track between trachea and esophagus. Feeding can cause coughing, cyanosis, and abdominal distension, due to air passing into the stomach; pulmonary fibrosis can be a later complication.

Transient tachypnea of the newborn

Other name Wet-lung disease

Transient tachypnea of the newborn is an increase in respiratory rate that can persist for about 24 h and then clear up. It is thought to be due to delayed clearance of fetal lung fluid after birth.

Treacher Collins syndrome

Treacher Collins syndrome is an autosomal dominant condition characterized mainly by maldevelopment of the facial skeleton. The mandible and malar bone are poorly developed and there are abnormalities of the external and middle ear, with hearing loss. The eyelids can be notched, and the eyelashes are poorly developed in the medial section of the lower lid. There is an antimongoloid slant of the eyes. Other features can be cleft palate, deficiencies of the fingers and toes, radioulnar synostosis, congenital heart disease, and narrowing of the pharynx. Death from respiratory infection is likely in the first month of life, but survivors of infancy can have a normal life span.

Tricho–dento–osseous syndrome

Other name T–D–O syndrome

Tricho–dento–osseous syndrome is an autosomal dominant disorder characterized by kinky hair, dolichocephaly, dental abnormalities, and sclerotic bones, and, sometimes, brittle nails and brown circular depressed areas of skin.

Tricho–rhino–phalangeal syndrome

Tricho–rhino–phalangeal syndrome appears in two forms:

(1) Fine brittle scalp hair, pear-shaped nose, abnormally short phalanges, small jaws, and dense medial half of the eyebrows.

(2) Sparse scalp hair, bulbous nose, microcephaly, abnormally short phalanges, large protruding ears, and mental retardation.

There is a partial deletion of chromosome 8q.

Tricuspid atresia

In tricuspid atresia, there is a failure of development of the right ventricular valve. There may be a ventricular septal defect which connects a large left ventricular chamber with a hypoplastic chamber representing the infundibulum of the right ventricle. An intra-atrial connection (usually a patent foramen) must be present if the child is to live. The great arteries may be normal or transposed, and there can be pulmonary stenosis or atresia. The incidence has been variously reported as between 1 in 18 000 and 1 in 30 000 live births.

See also Heart malformations

Tricuspid stenosis

Tricuspid stenosis can occur as a single lesion, without cyanosis, or in association with an underdeveloped right ventricle and an atrial septal defect, with cyanosis.

See also Heart malformations

Trismus pseudocamptodactyly syndrome
See Hecht syndrome

Trisomy 4p syndrome

Trisomy 4p syndrome is due to trisomy of part or most of the short arm of chromosome 4, and is characterized by growth deficiency of prenatal onset, severe mental retardation, an abnormal electroencephalogram, fits, a characteristic facies, additional or absent ribs, permanent flexion of some fingers, and other anomalies. About one-third of patients die in early infancy.

Trisomy 8 mosaic syndrome

Trisomy 8 syndrome in full is an early, lethal disorder. The majority of patients with trismomy 8 are mosaics. They are likely to be mentally retarded, and show a number of minor physical abnormalities, such as hypertelorism, strabismus, high-arched palate, permanent flexion of some fingers, a single palmar crease, vertebral anomalies, and agenesis of the corpus callosum.

Trisomy 9 mosaic syndrome

Trisomy 9 mosaic syndrome usually presents with congenital heart defects, joint contractures, a prominent upper lip covering the lower lip, low-set malformed ears, hypoplastic phalanges of the toes, and severe mental retardation. The majority of patients die in the postnatal period.

Trisomy 9p syndrome

Trisomy 9p syndrome is characterized by growth deficiency, mental retardation, delayed puberty, macrocephaly, hypertelorism, delayed closure of fontanels, and other anomalies.

Trisomy 13 syndrome
See Patau syndrome

Trisomy 21 syndrome
See Down syndrome

Truncus arteriosus

Truncus arteriosus is a heart malformation in which a single great artery arises from the heart to supply the pulmonary, systemic and coronary arteries. The incidence is about 1 in 33 000 live births. The atria and ventricles develop normally. The clinical presentation is usually with left-sided heart failure, cyanosis, and, sometimes, enlargement of the liver.

See also Heart malformations

Tuberous sclerosis

Other names Bourneville syndrome; Epiloia

Tuberous sclerosis is an autosomal dominant disorder characterized by fibrous–angiomatous lesions of the skin of the face, gliomatous and angiomatous tumors of the cortex, and white matter of the cerebral hemispheres, cyst-like areas in bone, angiomyolipomas of the kidney, convulsions, and severe mental retardation. Tumors can occur in other organs.

Turner syndrome

Other name Gonadal dysgenesis

Turner syndrome is one of the most common of chromosomal abnormalities. Frequency at conception is thought to be 1.5%, but most affected fetuses abort spontaneously, and the residual birth frequency is between 1 in 2500 and 1 in 3500. Common chromosomal abnormalities are 45,X0 sex chromosome karyotype (51%), mosaics of 45/46,XX sex chromosome (18%), and abnormal X chromosome structure (25%). Clinical features include low birth weight, lymphedema of the hands and feet at birth, low stature, obesity, incomplete development of the ovaries, incomplete development of secondary sexual characteristics, primary amenorrhea, low hairline, webbed or broad neck, hypoplastic nails, impaired hearing, an increased carrying angle at the elbows, short fourth metacarpal and metatarsal bones, pigmented nevi, aortic stenosis, and intestinal telangiectasia. Depression to a marked degree can be a complication.

Turner–Kieser syndrome
See Nail–patella syndrome

Tyrosinemia

Tyrosinemia is an increase in tyrosine in the blood and occurs in three forms – tyrosinema I, tyrosinemia II and transient neonatal tyrosinemia.

Tyrosinemia I is an autosomal recessive condition. It is rare except in people of French-Canadian descent. The primary cause is deficient activity of fumarylacetoacetate hydrolase. The acute form appears usually within the first 2 weeks of life, with severe liver disease, jaundice, hepatomegaly, bleeding, a progressive course, and death within the first or second year of life. The chronic type usually occurs in the second year with jaundice, hepatomegaly, abnormal liver function, neurological crises (pain, hypertonic posturing, paralysis), bleeding, liver failure, and death within 2–3 years.

Tyrosinemia II is a very rare autosomal recessive condition, characterized by mental retardation, keratitis, and painful hyperkeratotic lesions on the hands and feet.

Transient neonatal tyrosinemia is due to delayed maturation of parahydroxyphenylpyruvic acid oxidase. The blood tyrosine level is raised (the normal concentration is less than 120 μmol/l or 2.2 mg/dl) and there is an excessive excretion in the urine. It is more common in premature babies than full-term babies and in babies with a high protein intake (as occurs in babies fed on cow's milk). Vitamin C (ascorbic acid) reduces the tyrosine level. No physical abnormalities are present; mental retardation has been reported in some children with the condition.

U

Umbilical hernia

Umbilical hernia is a hernia through an orifice up to 4 cm in diameter in the umbilicus. The hernial sac is covered with skin and subcutaneous tissue (thus being different from an omphalocele) and can contain a loop of bowel, which is easily pushed back into the abdomen. It is most common in small babies. It occurs in 4% of white infants and 30% of black infants. A small hernia closes spontaneously.

Upper limb cardiovascular syndrome
See Lewis syndrome

Urachus lesions

The urachus is that remnant of the allantois that extends from the umbilicus to the bladder part of the cloaca. It may remain completely patent, with urine being discharged from the umbilicus. If the distal end does not obliterate, a drainage sinus results, with urine being discharged from it. Failure of obliteration of the proximal end results in a symptomless diverticulum of the bladder. Incomplete obliteration of the midportion causes the development of a urachal cyst, which can be obvious at birth or develop in infancy or childhood; the cyst frequently becomes infected.

Urea cycle disorders

Urea cycle disorders are due to a block in the urea cycle which is responsible for converting ammonium into urea. The six disorders are: N-acetylglutamate synthetase deficiency, carbamyl phosphate synthetase deficiency, ornithine transcarbamylase deficiency, citrullinemia, argininosuccinic acidemia, and, hyperargininemia

The first five of these produce severe symptoms in the 2nd or 3rd day of life: lethargy, hypotonia, fits, coma, hepatomegaly, and little or no liver function. A later version can develop in late infancy or early childhood. Hyperargininemia, which is due to deficiency of arginase, the final enzyme in the urea cycle, presents in childhood with spastic diplegia, ataxia and mental retardation.

Ureteric abnormalities

Megaureter

Megaureter is a widely dilated and often tortuous ureter. It can be due to obstruction or reflux, and some can occur without obstruction and reflux. In obstructive cases, the male:female ratio is 4:1; bilateral megaureter can occur. Non-obstructive, non-reflux megaureter can be associated with diabetes insipidus. Clinical features are likely to be urinary tract infection, pain, an abdominal mass, and hematuria.

Megacystis megaureter

Megacystis megaureter is characterized by dilated tortuous ureters, a large obstructed thin-walled bladder, and vesicoureteral reflux. The cause is unknown.

Duplicated ureters

Duplicated ureters can be complete or partial. A completely duplicated ureter is usually inserted into the normal position in the bladder, but it can open into an ectopic location in the urinary tract. They can be asymptomatic. They can be associated with obstruction, reflux, and ureterocele.

Ureterocele

Ureterocele is a cystic dilatation of the terminal, intravesical part of the ureter. It can be very small, or large enough to fill the bladder. It can be associated with duplicated ureters. Urinary tract infection is a complication.

Urethral valves

Urethral valves are flaps of tissue which occur in the anterior and posterior urethra, almost always in males. They can cause urinary obstruction, hydronephrosis and dysplasia of the kidneys with renal insufficiency.

Uridine diphosphate galactose-4-epimerase deficiency

Other name Epimerase deficiency

Uridine diphosphate galactose-4-epimerase deficiency is a rare condition in which there is an accumulation of galactose in blood and larger amounts of galactose-1-phosphate in red cells; epimerase activity in red cells is reduced. Usually, the condition is asymptomatic; jaundice, enlargement of the liver, and failure to thrive have been reported.

Usher syndrome

Usher syndrome is an association of retinitis pigmentosa with congenital sensorineural defect. It is usually an autosomal recessive condition with an incidence of 3.0–4.4 per 100 000.

Uvula abnormalities

Congenital cleft of the uvula occurs in 1 in 70 of the population. It varies from a small cleft of the tip, to a complete cleft. Associated conditions are a submucous cleft of the palate and insufficiency of the soft palate.

V

VACTEL syndrome

VACTEL syndrome is characterized by:
V – vertebral anomalies
A – anal anomalies
C – cardiac anomalies
TE – tracheoesophageal anomalies
L – limb anomalies

Van der Woude syndrome

Other name Lip pit–cleft lip syndrome

Van der Woude syndrome is an autosomal dominant condition in which there is an association of small pits in the lower lip with cleft lip. Other features can be cleft palate, cleft uvula, and absence of some teeth.

VATER syndrome

Vater syndrome is characterized by:
V – vertebral and cardiac ventricular defects
A – anal atresia
TE – tracheoesophageal fistula
R – radial and renal defects
Other defects can be pre- and postnatal growth deficiency, lower limb defects, external genitalia defects, and rib anomalies. There is also a single umbilical artery.

Velo-cardio-facial syndrome

Other name Shprintzen syndrome

Velo-cardio-facial syndrome is an autosomal dominant condition characterized by cleft palate, typical facies with a long face, retruded mandible, chin deficiency, abundant scalp hair, microcephaly (in about half the cases), conductive hearing loss, variable cardiovascular abnormalities (ventricular septal defect, tetralogy of Fallot, right aortic arch, abnormal left subclavian artery), short stature, hypotonia, slender limbs, hyperextensibility of fingers and toes, and slight mental retardation.

Vertebral body angioma

Congenital angioma of a vertebral body can cause collapse of a vertebra and compression of the spinal cord.

Vesicointestinal fissure
See Cloacal exstrophy (dystrophy)

Visceromegaly syndrome
See Beckwith–Wiedemann syndrome

Vitelline duct malformations

The vitelline duct (omphalomesenteric duct) connects the yolk sac with the midgut in the embryo through the umbilical cord; it should become obliterated and disappear. Rarely, it remains patent, in whole or in part. A patent duct presents with an enteroumbilical fistula, through which meconium and, later, feces are passed, and a loop of small bowel can be evaginated through the umbilical opening. A failure of the distal end of the duct to close produces a sinus, with the passage of a watery fluid from the umbilical cord and the presence of a red nodule at the base of the umbilicus. If the mid-portion of the duct persists, a cyst can form at the umbilicus.

Waardenburg–Klein syndrome
See Waardenburg syndrome

Waardenburg syndrome

Other names: Waardenburg–Klein syndrome; White forelock syndrome

Waardenburg syndrome is an autosomal dominant condition characterized by unilateral or bilateral sensorineural deafness, a white forelock, white eyebrows, a broad root of the nose, eyes of different colors, and patches of hypopigmentation of the skin. In type I, there is lateral displacement of the inner canthus; in type II, there is no displacement. There are *PAX3* gene mutations (2q). There can be an association with Hirschsprung disease.

WAGR syndrome

WAGR syndrome is characterized by:
W – Wilms tumor
A – aniridia
G – genital defects
R – retardation, mental

Walker–Warburg syndrome

Other name: HARD + E syndrome

Walker–Warburg syndrome is characterized by:
H – hydrocephalus
A – agyria
RD – retinal dysplasia
E – encephalocele
Death occurs within the first year of life.

Warburg syndrome

Warburg syndrome is an autosomal recessive condition characterized by defects of the brain and eyes. Cerebral defects are underdevelopment of some gyri and over-development of others, cerebellar hypoplasia, enlargement of the ventricles, and hydrocephalus.
Eye defects include microphthalmia, cataracts, coloboma, persistent
hyperplastic primary vitreous, and retinal dysplasia and detachment.
Most affected children die in the neonatal period. Survivors have
severe mental retardation.

Weaver syndrome

Weaver syndrome is characterized by accelerated growth and maturation beginning *in utero* and continuing after birth. In some cases,
the overgrowth begins a few months after birth. The head shows a
large bifrontal diameter and a flat occiput. Other features can be
hypertelorism, epicanthic folds, large ears, broad thumbs, permanent flexion of fingers, umbilical hernia and spasticity. The
male : female ratio is 3 : 1.

Weil–Marchesani syndrome

Weil–Marchesani syndrome is an autosomal recessive disorder of
connective tissue and is characterized by short stature, short fingers
and toes, stiff immobile joints, myopia, glaucoma, and dislocation of
the lens. Cardiac abnormalities may be present.

Wet-lung disease
See Transient tachypnea of the newborn

Whistling face syndrome
See Freeman–Sheldon syndrome

White forelock syndrome
See Waardenburg syndrome

Wiedemann–Beckwith syndrome

Wiedemann–Beckwith syndrome may be sporadic or an autosomal
dominant condition. It is characterized by exophthalmos, macroglossia, excessive growth postnatally, omphalocele or inguinal hernia,
and enlarged liver, pancreas, kidneys, and, sometimes, the heart.

Wiedemann–Raufenstrauch syndrome

Wiedemann–Raufenstrauch syndrome is probably an autosomal recessive condition. It is characterized by wide cranial sutures, a persistent anterior fontanel, sparse hair on the scalp, a small triangular face with a senile appearance, deep-set eyes, deficiency of subcutaneous fat, small size at birth, failure to thrive, and delayed motor and mental development.

Wildervanck syndrome

See Cervico–oculo–acoustic syndrome

Williams syndrome

Williams syndrome is a congenital condition occurring sporadically in which a high blood calcium level is associated with developmental delay, elfin facies, anteverted nostrils, strabismus, dental abnormalities, small nails, supravalvular aortic stenosis and other cardiovascular abnormalities, bladder diverticula, short stature, and mental retardation.

Williams–Beuren syndrome

Williams–Beuren syndrome occurs sporadically, but familial cases have been reported. The cause is unknown. Clinical features are facial dysmorphism, supravalvular aortic stenosis, hypercalcemia, and mental retardation.

Winchester syndrome

Other name Fibro-osteolytic dwarfism

Winchester syndrome is an autosomal recessive condition characterized by dwarfism, multiple contractures, joint destruction, corneal opacities, osteolysis of carpal and tarsal bones, osteoporosis, and gargoyle-like features.

Wiskott–Aldrich syndrome

Wiskott–Aldrich syndrome is an X-linked immunodeficiency due to a single locus defect on the short arm of the X chromosome. Affected boys have small abnormal platelets and severe thrombocytopenia. Clinical features are eczema, recurrent infections and hemorrhages, and, rarely, malignancies of the lymphoreticular system. Death is usual under 10 years of age.

Wolf-Hirschhorn syndrome

See Chromosome 4, short-arm deletion syndrome

X-linked agammaglobulinemia

X-linked agammaglobulinemia is a congenital antibody deficiency disease, due to a failure of B-cell development, usually at the stage of pre-B cells. There is a defect in a single locus on the long arm of the X chromosome. The disease has a frequency of 1 in 50 000 to 1 in 100 000. Affected males present in infancy or early childhood with recurrent pyogenic infections. There is a severe deficiency of circulating B cells; plasma cells are absent from lymph nodes and bone marrow; pre-B cells are found in the bone marrow. Some patients have near-normal numbers of immature B cells in the peripheral circulation.

X-linked chronic granulomatous disease

X-linked chronic granulomatous disease is a rare form of immunodeficiency. The gene is carried on the short arm of the X chromosome. It is an inherited disorder of phagocyte function, due to defective production of superoxide. A phenotypically identical disease is inherited as an autosomal recessive gene.

X-linked ichthyosis

X-linked ichthyosis is a skin disorder which occurs only in males. It is associated with deficiency of steroid sulfatase. Clinical features are ichthyotic scales, corneal dystrophy, and cryptorchidism (in 25%).

X-linked immunodeficiency

Six human immunodeficiency diseases are associated with the X chromosome. They are: severe combined immunodeficiency, Wiskott–Aldrich syndrome, X-linked agammaglobulinemia, X-linked antibody deficiency with hyper-IgM, X-linked chronic granulomatous disease, and X-linked lymphoproliferative syndrome.

Genetic mapping with restriction fragment length polymorphisms has assigned these diseases to specific loci on the X chromosome. Lyon's hypothesis asserts that these X-linked immunodeficiencies may be detectable in carriers of the diseases as a result of X-chromosome inactivation of the normal disease gene. Genetic mapping allows probability-based prenatal diagnosis.

X-linked immunodeficiency with hyper-IgM

X-linked immunodeficiency with hyper-IgM appears to be due to a single defect on the long arm of the X chromosome; the gene responsible has been assigned to Xq24–27. It has been associated with the presence of B cells with surface immunoglobulins of only the IgM and IgD isotypes and the presence of elevated levels of IgM and/or IgD in the serum. Clinical features are likely to be respiratory infections, otitis, diarrhea, and oral ulcers.

X-linked hydrocephalus syndrome

X-linked hydrocephalus syndrome is an X-linked recessive syndrome characterized by the development of hydrocephalus *in utero*, spasticity, stenosis of the cerebral aqueduct, short flexed thumbs, and mental retardation. Other features can be an abnormal electroencephalogram, fits, absence of the corpus callosum, and other brain defects.

X-linked lymphoproliferative syndrome

X-linked lymphoproliferative syndrome is an X-linked immunodeficiency with a defect in a single locus on the long arm of the X chromosome. There is an abnormal immune response to Epstein–Barr virus, and the syndrome becomes manifest after infection with the virus. The disease is manifested by a severe and often fatal mononucleosis and acquired immunodeficiency. The mean age at presentation is 5 years. Clinical features are fever, raised white-cell count, atypical lymphocytes, hemorrhage, jaundice, hepatic necrosis and failure, with death after an illness of 2–3 weeks.

X-linked severe combined immunodeficiency

X-linked severe combined immunodeficiency is a phenotypic term applied to infants who have a severe deficiency of T cells, and, in some infants, of B cells. It is inherited as an autosomal recessive or an X-linked condition. In about half the infants with an autosomal recessive inheritance, there is an inherited deficiency of one of the purine degradation enzymes, adenosine deaminase or purine nucleoside phosphorylase; and other rarer causes of these conditions can be deficiency of interleukin-2, of CD3, or of the phosphatidyl inositol pathway of T-cell activation. The incidence is $1:1\,000\,000$ to $1:500\,000$. The male:female ratio is about $3:1$. The infants, in addition to having a severe deficiency of T cells, have severely compromised cell-mediated immunity, fail to thrive, have severe opportunistic infections, and usually die in infancy.

X-linked spondyloepiphyseal dysplasia tarda

Other name Spondyloepiphyseal dysplasia tarda

X-linked spondyloepiphyseal dysplasia tarda is characterized by short stature, flattened vertebrae with a central 'hump' in the region of their epiphyses, small iliac wings of the pelvis, short femoral neck, with osteoarthritis developing in adult life.

XXX syndrome

In triple X syndrome, abnormalities are slight. The ovaries are often normal and the patient is fertile. Intelligence may be impaired and there may be behavioral problems.

XXXX syndrome

XXXX syndrome is characterized by mental retardation, behavioral and speech problems, and various physical abnormalities, such as mid-facial hypoplasia, hypertelorism, epicanthic folds, radioulnar synostosis, and fifth finger clinodactyly.

XXXXX syndrome

Other name Penta X syndrome

XXXXX syndrome is characterized by mental retardation, growth deficiency, microcephaly, mongoloid eyes, low nasal bridge, hypertelorism, epicanthic folds, patent ductus arteriosus, small hands, incurved fifth fingers, and failure to thrive. Other features can be multiple joint dislocations, renal dysplasia, overlapping toes, low-set ears, coloboma of the iris, simian creases, and equinovarus.

XXXY and XXXXY syndromes

XXXY and XXXXY syndromes are characterized by short stature, retarded bony maturation, wide-set eyes, strabismus, low nasal bridge, prognathism, abnormal ears, short neck, minor limb abnormalities, cryptorchidism, small penis, and mental retardation.

XXY syndrome

See Klinefelter syndrome

XYY syndrome

XYY syndrome is characterized by tall stature and aberrant behavior. The incidence is 1 in 840 newborn male children. Clinical features are likely to be accelerated growth after the age of 5 or 6 years, poor development of pectoral and shoulder girdle muscles, poor motor coordination, acne, aggressive behavior, temper tantrums, and mental retardation. The features in some people are slight and the chromosomal abnormality may not be detected.

Z

Zellweger syndrome

Other name Cerebro-hepato-renal syndrome

Zellweger syndrome is an inherited (probably autosomal recessive) syndrome characterized by imperfect myelinization of nerve tracts, microgyria, calcific deposits in long bones, craniofacial malformations, hypospadias, glaucoma, cataracts, renal cysts, enlarged liver, hyperbilirubinemia, extramedullary hemopoiesis, and hypotonia. There is a reduction in the amount of dihydroacetate phosphate acetyltransferase (DHAP-AT) and an absence of hepatic and renal peroxisomes. Death occurs in infancy.

Zerres-Rietschel syndrome

Zerres-Rietschel syndrome is characterized by multiple congenital abnormalities, including microcephaly, dysmorphic facies, short stature, syndactyly, hearing defect, and mental retardation.

Zinsser-Engmann syndrome

Other name Dyskeratosis congenita

Zinsser-Engmann syndrome may be present at birth, but usually appears later. Clinical features are leukoplakia of the conjunctival, genital and urethral mucosa, reticulate hyperpigmentation of the skin, usually on the neck, upper chest and upper arms, nail dystrophy, osteoporosis, avascular necrosis of bone, and fractures. The inheritance is uncertain.